MEN UNDER PRESSURE

MEN
UNDER
PRESSURE

A MAN'S GUIDE TO RECLAIMING MENTAL HEALTH

WHITNEY WRIGHT

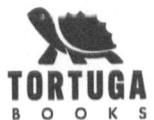

TORTUGA
BOOKS

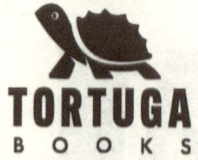

TORTUGA
B O O K S

MEN UNDER PRESSURE
A Man's Guide to Reclaiming Mental Health
First Edition

Published by Tortuga Books

ISBN   979-8-9925378-0-2   *Hardcover*
       979-8-9925378-1-9   *Paperback*
       979-8-9925378-2-6   *Ebook*

Cover and interior design by John van der Woude, JVDW Designs.

For more information about the book or to contact the author, visit *www.menunderpressure.com*.

The information provided in this book is for informational purposes only and should not be construed as professional or medical advice on any subject matter. This book is not intended to be a substitute for professional medical advice, diagnosis, or treatment. While the author has made every effort to ensure accuracy, readers should always consult with qualified healthcare professionals before making any decisions based on the content within. The publisher and author disclaim any liability for any losses, damages, or risks arising, directly or indirectly, from the use and application of any of the contents of this work.

If you are in crisis or you think you may have an emergency, call your doctor or 911 immediately. If you're having suicidal thoughts, call 1-800-273-TALK (8255) to talk to a skilled, trained counselor at a crisis center in your area at any time (National Suicide Prevention Lifeline). If you are located outside the United States, call your local emergency line immediately.

For Margaret and our three incredible kids

And to all the men out there struggling to keep their heads above water. I've been there and done that, and I'm so done with that.

CONTENTS

PART THREE. UP TO MY NECK

PART FOUR. DIVING DEEP

FOREWORD

by Dr. Brett Kessler
President of the American Dental Association

Let me start by saying this: I was once a dentist with a serious struggle—I was in an absolute love affair with cocaine. The pressures of dentistry, coupled with my own unaddressed addictions, nearly destroyed my life.

But before I dive into that part of my story, let me tell you about meeting Dr. Whitney Wright.

I graduated in 1995 from the University of Illinois Chicago College of Dentistry with big dreams and the drive to succeed. Afterward, I moved to Michigan with my wife, who was beginning her orthodontic residency. While she focused on her training, I threw myself into my career, balancing private practice with teaching at the dental school. It seemed like I was on the perfect path—but appearances can be deceiving. Beneath the surface, I was battling demons that would soon threaten to destroy everything I'd built.

By 2005, I was working part-time as a faculty member at the University of Colorado School of Dental Medicine. Whitney was just beginning to treat patients, and he stood out right away. He had this way of laughing and joking with patients that put them completely at ease, effortlessly switching between English and Spanish. I enjoyed watching him grow more confident in the clinic. When he asked to visit my private practice in Stapleton, Colorado, I agreed. I could tell he was eager to understand what life as a dentist was really like.

The day he visited my office, Whitney was brimming with questions—not just about dentistry but about life. We discovered we shared a passion for cycling, and I even showed him the triathlon bike I was planning to buy at the time. After a few hours of conversation about balancing work and personal life, he left with an unmistakable excitement about his future in the field. I admired his energy and enthusiasm. Little did I know both of us would face incredible challenges in the years to come.

I eventually left the university to focus on my private practice, and I wouldn't cross paths with Whitney again for nearly two decades. By 2023, my life had taken me in unexpected directions. I was now the chairman of the Well-Being Advisory Committee for the American Dental Association (ADA), a role born from my own battles with addiction and mental health. Several years earlier, the ADA had launched a campaign to support dentists struggling with these issues, offering resources to help them recover. It was through this initiative that Whitney and I reconnected.

We invited him to participate in the ADA's well-being program after we learned about his own struggles. I was in charge of the interview process, so we met for lunch in Denver.

I'll never forget our conversation.

Whitney opened up about his journey after dental school, the pressures of building a dental and orthodontic company, and how those pressures eventually broke him. He was brutally honest—unflinchingly so—sharing personal traumas that laid the foundation for his struggles. His openness impressed me, and his deep desire to help other dentists *inspired* me. Here was someone who, like me, had risen from the rubble and was determined to make a difference.

The dental profession has long been associated with elevated suicide rates. While recent studies offer a more nuanced perspective, there's no denying the pressures of this career. Dentistry demands precision, compassion, and resilience. Small errors can carry severe repercussions, and many dentists work in private practices, isolated from larger support networks. The physical strain of long hours, the financial burden of student loans and running a practice, and the mental toll of trying to meet patients' expectations can feel overwhelming. Add to this the stigma surrounding mental health in our profession, and it's no wonder so many dentists feel trapped. I know I did.

My own battle with addiction started when I was nineteen, long before dental school. At first, it was just part of the party scene—marijuana, mushrooms, acid—but it quickly escalated to cocaine. By the time I began practicing, addiction had controlled my life for more than ten years. I went on binges, consuming everything I could until it was gone. I hid it well, but the cracks were showing.

My long-lasting disguise came off during a work trip. I had taken my Michigan staff to a continuing education course in Chicago but abandoned them at the hotel after buying a lot of cocaine. I went on a three-day binge, leaving them stranded in an unfamiliar city. I missed the course entirely, and when I returned, my team had questions I couldn't dodge. That was my wake-up call. I entered a six-week rehab program for the first time, but sobriety didn't come immediately. I continued to relapse, and it wasn't until a year and a half later when I hit my ultimate low: I missed my best friend's mother's funeral because I was on another binge. That was the moment I decided I was done.

Recovery wasn't easy. My wife stood by me, but she also held me accountable. She made an appointment for me to return to rehab and left me alone for a few days to figure it out. Her support—and her boundaries—pushed me to confront my addiction head-on. When we moved to Colorado in 1999, I disclosed my addiction history while applying for my dental license. That honesty led to professional challenges: I couldn't get liability insurance, disability insurance, or life insurance. The Colorado Dental Board placed me on probation, requiring random drug tests, therapy, and practice monitoring. At the time, it felt like punishment, but in hindsight, it was exactly what I needed.

These monitoring programs are often misunderstood as punitive, but they're lifesaving. The program I entered had a 75 percent success rate compared to the 3–6 percent success rate of those trying to recover alone. I was forced to engage in positive behaviors like regular therapy, monitored sobriety, and accountability measures. While it was grueling at the time, it worked. Over three years, I built a track record of sobriety and excellence in my practice, proving to myself and others that I was more than my addiction.

Eventually, I found the courage to share my story publicly. It took years to shed the shame, but when I did, I discovered the power of my voice. I became the chair of Colorado's dental well-being program, personally answering phone calls from dentists hitting their own rock bottoms and contemplating suicide. It was humbling, and it gave my struggles purpose.

Today, as president of the ADA, I've made it my mission to reduce the stigma around mental health and addiction in healthcare. We're working to eliminate discriminatory questions from licensure renewals and insurance applications, ensuring that professionals can seek help without fear of judgment or career repercussions.

I can't help but think about how much I would have benefited from a book like Whitney's *Men Under Pressure* during my darkest days. His courage in sharing his story has the power to save lives—not just the lives of dentists, but of every single man weighed down by the pressures they face in their lives today.

I'm grateful to have played a small part in his journey. Together, we're proving that recovery is possible and that no one has to face their struggles alone.

—Brett Kessler, DDS

INTRODUCTION

There I was, thirty-six years old, hyperventilating, drenched in sweat, alternating between vomiting into the toilet and curling up in the fetal position on the cold floor of the restroom of my orthodontic office. I was in the throes of a severe panic attack, and it wasn't my first. My mental health had been unraveling for some time, but I kept telling myself that a "real man" doesn't show weakness. He doesn't show fear. He's supposed to be the immovable pillar of strength, the rock that others rely on in life's storm.

But I was crumbling. Hard. Sobs racked my body as the panic attack intensified, reaching a terrifying crescendo.

How did I end up here?

What could I have done differently?

How do I recover from this?

Will I lose everything I've worked so hard for?

Am I a failure for even showing cracks in my armor?

Who am I?

In my personal life, I'm a family man. My wife, Margaret, and I have been married for over twenty years, and we have three wonderful children. Professionally, I'm the founding orthodontist (and former chief clinical officer) of a dental company that now spans twenty-seven offices across four states, employing 100 dentists and 850 staff members. Our company, Risas Dental and Braces, has won numerous awards since we opened our doors in Arizona in 2011. As of 2024, we've treated over 750,000 patients, received 25,000 five-star reviews, and given away more than $11 million in free dental care to our community. With more than 3.8 million patient visits, I'm incredibly proud of what Risas has become.

But it hasn't come without a personal cost. Building this company has been a journey filled with literal blood, sweat, and tears. And behind all the success, I was terrified of falling apart—both personally and professionally—because of my mental health.

In 2016, five years after we launched, the panic attacks began. At the time, I didn't realize these episodes would mark the start of a life-altering journey. I wasn't just going to be dipping my toes into the waters of mental health—I was diving headfirst into its dark, murky depths.

If you or someone you love is struggling, let me be the first to say this: There is hope. It does get better.

If you're suffering, too, I want you to know that I see you. And I want for you the same thing you likely want for yourself: to get better. Not all of you will want or need to dive as deep as I had to in order to heal, and that's okay. In this book, I'll offer tips on how to gently wade into those waters—or how to strap on a scuba tank and dive deep, depending on where you are in your own life.

For me, I didn't have a choice—I *had* to dive deep. In fact, a few years after the attacks began, my psychiatrist told me, "Whitney, you need to heal, or you will die. For now, it's just panic attacks. Soon it'll be heart attacks."

Shortly after that conversation, I checked myself into Sierra Tucson, a rehabilitation facility in Southern Arizona, for thirty days.

MEN AND MENTAL HEALTH

Data from the National Institute of Mental Health show that approximately one in five adult men in the United States, or about 20 percent of the adult male population, experiences a mental health challenge each year. Despite the significant prevalence of mental health issues, only about 35–45 percent of these men actively seek help. A substantial portion of men don't pursue treatment due to stigma, societal expectations, or a lack of awareness about mental health issues.[1]

But *why*? When it comes to mental health, it can feel like pulling teeth to get men to crack open *that* Pandora's Box (and I know a thing or two about pulling teeth). Who wants to dive into the depths of their emotions and confront their demons? I sure didn't.

But just like a toothache, ignoring our mental health only makes things worse. I've got the emotional scars to prove it.

For example, my name is Dr. *Whitney* Wright. The name is misleading—I'm a guy. I know that previous statement may stir up some discontent among those who feel that names shouldn't have a gender, but I grew up in the eighties, when they certainly did. And I was ridiculed for having a girl's name.

There's a "Dr." in front of my name, too. However, I'm not a psychiatrist, psychologist, or certified therapist—I'm an ortho-dontist—though after everything I've experienced, I often feel like one. I consider myself a mental health advocate, but I didn't learn about mental disorders in a classroom. Instead, I learned through personal experience, having developed, lived with, and ultimately learned strategies to help me navigate these challenges and heal.

My journey into mental health awareness began when severe anxiety and depression forced me to permanently stop putting braces in faces just five short years after becoming an orthodontist. This initial awareness led me to discover the different issues I've had to deal with in my lifetime:

- Toxic shame
- Codependency
- Attention deficit hyperactivity disorder (ADHD)
- Destructive coping mechanisms
- Post-traumatic stress disorder (PTSD)
- Adrenal fatigue
- Depression
- Anxiety
- Burnout

While this might seem like a daunting list of issues—and trust me, it is—I aim to share what these things are, how I developed them, the toll they took on me, and the steps I took to reclaim my life from their destructive grip. I'll describe each disorder as I share my story with the hope it may help you identify similar feelings you might be experiencing and begin the road to recovery.

You might be wondering why I'd choose to reveal my vulnerabilities. Why would I want to expose the mental struggles that have caused me so much guilt, shame, and pain? The answer is simple: *I hope that by sharing my story, you can avoid the suffering I endured—or, if you're past the point of avoiding it, that you may see a light at the end of whatever tunnel of suffering you may be facing now.*

In this book, I'll take you on my life's journey, sharing the experiences that have shaped my understanding of mental health and the lessons I've learned along the way. We'll explore the highs and lows, the triumphs and failures, and the moments that forced me to confront my own mental well-being. But this isn't just my story; it's a roadmap for anyone struggling with mental health issues, especially men who often feel the need to suffer in silence.

Together in this book, we'll explore the science behind mental health disorders and examine how they develop and manifest in our lives. As I share my own experiences with depression, anxiety, PTSD, burnout, and more, you may recognize similar symptoms in your own life and feel encouraged to seek help. More importantly, I'll illustrate that there is hope and that recovery is possible, no matter how dark things may seem. This book also includes stories from other "Men Under Pressure" who have opened up to me about their mental health struggles. With their permission, I've shared their stories. They hope that by sharing their experiences, they can help men who feel alone and overwhelmed realize they aren't isolated in their struggles. Their stories are real and truly inspirational.

We'll tackle some heavy topics, but I promise to include some funny stories and moments of comic relief when things get intense. While I may appear lighthearted, I've faced serious pain, just like many of you. My goal is to foster open and honest conversations about mental health, particularly for men who often feel compelled to put on a brave face and suffer in silence.

FOR THOSE WHO LOVE MEN UNDER PRESSURE

This book is primarily for men, but if you're the spouse or family member of a man who's struggling, you've come to the right place.

There may be answers in here for him, and one method to encourage him to read it might be with a simple invitation, something like, "Hey, sweetheart, check out this book that shows how this guy with a girl's name became successful and then crashed and burned, hard. It's crazy how he pulled himself up from the abyss. Some parts of it reminded me of some of the things you may be dealing with, and I thought you may want to read it."

Then just leave it on his nightstand. Hopefully, he'll pick it up and find something that helps him be a happier, healthier, less stressed man. Men, if your wife pulled this on you, you can blame me...now keep reading, buddy. (Note that when I say "wife," I also mean girlfriend, boyfriend, husband, life partner, mother, or any other iteration of a loving relationship you may be in, so please don't cancel me.)

Women, my intent is to show you that you can positively impact a man in your life who's struggling by allowing him to open up and "be vulnerable," as Dr. Brené Brown suggests, discussing what affects his life. As previously mentioned, men are often terrified of failing and letting others down, especially those who count on them.

I remember the first time I finally truly opened up to my wife, Margaret, about what was happening beneath the surface. I was terrified that she was going to be disgusted with her choice of a mate and immediately leave me for some handsome, tatted-up, ripped alpha male straight off the cover of a romance novel who would never have such weaknesses or insecurities.

To my immense relief, my tear-filled words were met with grace and a gentle understanding so profound that I wept like a child. In that moment, the feelings of pure love and acceptance I'd been yearning for flooded into my heart.

To be clear, she'd never withheld those emotions from me. It was my own shame, guilt, and fear that had blocked me from allowing myself to feel them. I cannot begin to convey the enormity of that moment. I'll forever be grateful for her unwavering support and love during some of the most challenging times of my life. Our relationship has never been stronger.

Thank you, Margaret. You are not only my best friend—you are, without a doubt, the love of my life.

So, ladies, I wholeheartedly believe that when a man opens up to you, you'll support him and encourage future open and honest dialogue. He may expect revulsion, anger, fear, or contempt at what he shares. Instead, he'll receive love, compassion, empathy, and kindness. You may need to just hold him and let him cry if he needs to. After we're done blubbering for a bit, we'll pick ourselves back up, feeling lighter, stronger, and loved more deeply than we ever thought possible. Sometimes, we just need to let off some steam.

WHAT'S NEXT?

It's time to settle in, grab a snack, and get ready to break down the stigma surrounding mental health.

(I've heard from reliable sources that four out of five dentists recommend snacking on something that won't mess up your teeth. Don't choose corn nuts. My childhood dentist once joked that corn nuts helped put his kids through college. And what's up with that fifth dentist? It seems like they just want to see the world burn.)

Together we'll explore practical strategies for managing the pressures of everyday life, reducing stress and anxiety, and addressing various mental health conditions—all while discovering the power of vulnerability and self-acceptance. To accomplish this, I've divided this book into four main parts:

- **Part One: Building Pressure**—My story and how I ended up being blown to smithereens
- **Part Two: Wading In**—Ways to help yourself heal on your own
- **Part Three: Up to My Neck**—Getting professional help if you need to wade deeper into murky waters
- **Part Four: Diving Deep**—Severe cases require severe treatment. How thirty days in an inpatient facility saved me and many other men

In **Appendix A**,[2] you'll find questionnaires you can take on your own to help you better understand your own relationship with deep topics such as toxic shame, childhood trauma, codependency, unhealthy coping mechanisms, ADHD, PTSD, adrenal fatigue, depression, anxiety, burnout, and addiction.

In **Appendix B**, you'll find a list of recommended reading if any of these topics inspire you to explore further. My ultimate goal is that by the end of our time together, you'll have the tools and knowledge to prioritize your mental well-being and build a life that brings you joy, both on the surface and deep within. Taking care of your mental health doesn't make you weak, guys; it makes you a well-balanced human being. If a Type-A, workaholic orthodontist—who is deeply concerned about maintaining his professional credibility—can learn to embrace his traumas, fears, and emotions and emerge stronger, then so can you.

Remember that if you or someone you know is struggling, there is help and hope available. To anyone trapped in a pit of despair, know that escape is possible. Life can improve! So, if you'll allow me to share my journey—a rise to success followed by a significant fall into disability—perhaps you'll learn something that can help you navigate your own challenges and lead a healthier and happier life.

Alright, that's enough of that. Now, let's get back to the story.

(I encourage you to reread those last two sentences in the voice of the late Peter Falk, the actor who portrayed the book-reading grandfather in the eighties cult classic *The Princess Bride*. If you haven't seen that movie, do yourself a favor and watch it—preferably with your loved ones.)

Thank you for indulging me. I'm all sorts of weird.

So, without further ado, let's proceed.

GET THE

MEN UNDER PRESSURE
WORKBOOK

TAKE THIS JOURNEY EVEN DEEPER

This book isn't just about reading—it's about
action. The *Men Under Pressure* workbook
is designed to help you reflect, process, and
apply what you're learning with guided
prompts and exercises for each chapter.

Get your free workbook now:
Scan the QR code or
visit *workbook.menunderpressure.com*

CHANGE STARTS HERE.

PART ONE
BUILDING PRESSURE

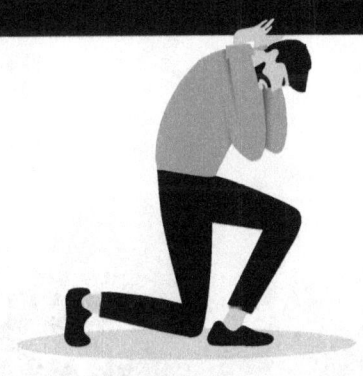

WHY ARE MEN UNDER PRESSURE?

Stay calm. Be sure to smile. They said this place was the best, I told myself as I checked into Sierra Tucson, a well-known mental health rehab facility. *So it must be okay. Breathe. Get through it.*

My road here had been a long one: By ignoring the red flags, pushing past my limits, and avoiding the demons of my past, I'd nearly destroyed myself. My psychiatrist had recommended this facility as the best option to piece my life back together. I'd be lying if I said I wasn't terrified of dropping everything—leaving my beloved wife and children, along with all my responsibilities, to check in. And yet, here I was.

In the back of my mind, one nagging question remained: *How did I get here?*

THE PRESSURE TO BE A HUSBAND

Men today face tremendous pressures from all sorts of unrealistic societal expectations that often coincide with traditional roles—roles that come with deeply ingrained responsibilities. This dynamic can lead to overwhelming feelings of stress, particularly as we feel the constant need to uphold ideals of strength, stability, and competence. One of those roles, as I've known them, is that of a partner.

I've been married for twenty-two years now, and as husbands, I know we're often expected to provide unwavering support. Society traditionally casts men as the "rock" in the relationship—the steady force that must remain composed and strong, even during times of crisis. This can create silent pressure that can leave men feeling as if they cannot express their vulnerabilities or emotions openly for fear that exposing weakness will be the beginning of the end. In relationships, this often leads to emotional suppression, which can result in disconnected communication, pent-up frustration, or even mental health issues like anxiety and depression. Despite the changing dynamics in gender roles, many men still feel compelled to uphold a traditional sense of masculinity within their marriages, fearing that vulnerability may be perceived as weakness.

FATHERHOOD AND THE EXPECTATION OF LEADERSHIP

Fatherhood comes with its own unique pressures. As a father of three wonderful kids, I know that men are traditionally expected to be role models, providers, and protectors for their children. In modern society, the father figure is often seen as a crucial necessity to a child's development—particularly for sons, who look to their fathers to learn how to navigate manhood. Fathers are frequently tasked with teaching discipline, responsibility, and values while also being emotionally available and nurturing to their children. Striking this balance can be challenging, as many men don't express their emotions freely. The expectation to "lead by example" while maintaining authority in the household can be daunting, especially as they navigate their own internal struggles or societal pressures.

FINANCIAL PRESSURES AND THE ROLE OF PROVIDER

The expectation that men should be the primary financial providers continues to be a dominant narrative in many cultures. Even as an early teen, I frequently worried about how I would provide for my future family. Not too long ago, my teenage son expressed he was struggling with those exact same worries. I believe this is very typical among men growing up, even from an early age. In spite of the growing number of dual-income households, societal pressures around providing for one's family remain deeply embedded. Men are often measured by their financial success and their ability to sustain a stable home life. The fear of financial instability or failure to meet these expectations can create intense stress and anxiety. Men may also feel pressure to continuously "level up" in their careers, leading to a work-life imbalance that can strain relationships, cause

burnout, and affect mental health. For some, the financial burden is coupled with the fear of losing their identity or worth if
they cannot fulfill their roles as providers. I definitely fell into
this last category, and it was brutal.

BEING A PILLAR OF STRENGTH IN THE COMMUNITY

Some men feel compelled to be pillars of strength in their communities. I've felt this same pressure. While I was building my
company, I was asked to serve for five years as the bishop (or
minister) of my congregation of more than 400 members. Being
responsible for the spiritual, emotional, and financial welfare
of an entire congregation was a daunting task. This expectation
to constantly perform at high levels in the public sphere can
lead to feelings of isolation, as men may not feel they can show
weakness or ask for help without diminishing their standing in
the community.

THE BURDEN OF EMOTIONAL STOICISM

Across all these roles—husband, father, provider, and community leader—men are frequently expected to maintain emotional stoicism. The deeply ingrained societal belief that "real
men don't cry" or show vulnerability often leads men to suppress their emotions, further amplifying stress and anxiety.
This is exactly what happened to me. I was terrified of showing my weaknesses to anybody, especially my family. By hiding
what was really happening beneath a fake calm surface, the

turbulent waters I concealed beneath eroded my long-term stability. Emotional suppression can have detrimental effects on mental health, contributing to higher rates of depression, substance abuse, and even suicide among men. The pressure to "hold it together" for our families and communities can lead to a mental and emotional breaking point, as men are often left feeling unsupported and unable to express their struggles openly.

■ ■ ■

The pressures men face in all these different roles can be both emotionally and mentally taxing. The expectations to be strong, successful, and unshakeable in the face of adversity are often unrealistic and unsustainable. Encouraging men to embrace vulnerability, seek help when needed, and balance societal expectations with their personal needs is crucial for fostering healthier mental and emotional well-being. And, if you don't know by now, that's exactly what I'm here to help you with.

THE NEED FOR PRESSURE

Let me be clear: Pressure in and of itself isn't necessarily a bad thing. I like to think of men as old-fashioned steam locomotives. A steam locomotive operates by burning fuel in a firebox to heat water in a large boiler, generating steam. As the steam builds pressure, the train driver, or locomotive engineer, adjusts knobs and pulls levers to direct the pressure, driving pistons that turn the wheels. When enough pressure is gathered, the conductor can guide the locomotive to its destination.

I've witnessed incredible things when men effectively balance their inner fire with their external pressures. Without a fair amount of pressure in the boiler, though, that train can become stagnant, regardless of how fiercely the fire burns. That's why I believe pressure can ultimately help us reach our goals, if only we know the right kind of pressure to leverage and how to take care of ourselves while we do it.

Traditionally, directly behind the locomotive is the tender or "coal car." The tender holds both fuel for the fire and additional water for the boiler. As we strive to balance stoking our fire with managing the boiler's pressure, we may need to make adjustments to keep our train running smoothly. In the early days of steam locomotives, wood was the primary fuel. As technology advanced, coal and oil became preferred for their hotter, longer burn. If the fire isn't hot enough or lacks sufficient fuel, the engine won't generate enough pressure to create momentum. Conversely, if the fire receives too much fuel and burns too hot, it can lead to serious consequences. One possibility is running out of fuel before reaching the destination, which I would liken to burnout. When we exhaust our resources too quickly, we may find ourselves stranded, wondering how our fire went cold. The other scenario involves dangerously high internal pressure, which could cause the locomotive to explode. Sadly, I've experienced both burnout and explosion.

Inside the locomotive's cab is a critical safety valve. When opened, it vents excess steam and maintains safe pressure levels. If this valve isn't opened when pressure rises—*KABOOM*—the boiler explodes! If the engineer is too preoccupied with passenger comfort, overly concerned about the food and beverage car, or stressed over baggage organization, he might miss the warning signs of climbing pressure.

In my life, I failed to balance my pressures effectively. I got distracted by numerous responsibilities, ignored the warning signs, and ultimately had a meltdown. When driving our metaphorical locomotive, if we don't occasionally open the safety valve to "let off steam," the boiler can blow, bringing the entire train to a halt. Such an explosion can cause severe harm and lasting damage, which is truly devastating.

STIGMA SURROUNDING MEN'S MENTAL HEALTH

Before we can dive into the murky waters of self-healing, we need to discuss the elephant in the room: stigma. One of the massive hurdles that stands in the way of men getting better is the negative stigma they face when they attempt to fight their demons. It's the epitome of being trapped between a rock and a hard place. They want to get better, but they don't want to face the backlash of opening up about it. Stigma refers to a set of negative beliefs, attitudes, or prejudices that society holds toward a particular group, condition, or behavior. Sadly, it often leads to discrimination, marginalization, or exclusion, and it can significantly impact those targeted. This societal judgment can deter people from seeking help or disclosing their struggles, fearing they'll be seen as "weak" or "unstable."

It's estimated that around 60 percent of middle-aged men with mental health challenges remain undiagnosed, a statistic often attributed to a reluctance to seek help, societal stigma surrounding mental health, and the tendency for men to minimize or ignore their symptoms. Furthermore, misdiagnosis is a significant concern in mental health care; studies suggest that about 15–30 percent of middle-aged men may be misdiagnosed when they do seek help. This misdiagnosis can stem from gender biases in diagnosis, overlapping symptoms with other conditions, or inadequate screening.[3]

Men face unique stigmas when it comes to mental health, which are often rooted in traditional views of masculinity. Ultimately, I found the more I opened up about the issues I was facing, the weaker their grip on me became. Common stigmas men encounter include:

1. **Weakness or Incompetence**: Many men fear that admitting to mental health issues is a sign of weakness or incompetence. This is particularly damaging because traditional masculinity values emotional control and strength. Men are often expected to "man up" and suppress their emotions, leading to a reluctance to acknowledge feelings of anxiety, depression, or burnout.

2. **Fear of Losing Status**: Men, especially those in positions of authority, may fear that revealing mental health struggles will cost them respect among peers, colleagues, or family members. The societal notion that mental illness diminishes one's capability to lead or succeed discourages many men from seeking help.

3. **Association with Femininity**: Mental health treatment is sometimes seen as a "feminine" activity, further perpetuating the stigma for men. Emotional vulnerability, seeking therapy, or expressing feelings is often considered incompatible with the ideals of masculinity, which prize independence and toughness.

4. **Failure as a Provider**: Since men are often seen as primary providers and protectors, there's a stigma attached to mental health issues that implies men are failing in their responsibilities. The pressure to maintain the appearance of being a capable husband, father, and provider exacerbates their reluctance to admit when they need help.

OVERCOMING THE STIGMA

Efforts to overcome mental health stigma are gaining momentum through increased awareness, changing societal norms, and advocacy. Public awareness campaigns, like those from the Movember Foundation and the National Alliance on Mental Illness (NAMI), encourage men to talk openly about their mental health, helping to normalize these conversations. Celebrities and professional athletes such as Dwayne "The Rock" Johnson, Jim Carrey, Kevin Love, and Michael Phelps have shared their struggles, demonstrating that mental health issues can affect anyone, regardless of status.

Many workplaces are also stepping up, offering employee assistance programs and mental health days to create safe environments for discussion. Additionally, cultural narratives around masculinity are shifting, with more men embracing vulnerability and redefining strength as the ability to seek help. To that end, some mental health professionals are tailoring therapy specifically for men, focusing on practical, action-oriented approaches that resonate with traditional male socialization, which has been invaluable in my own healing journey with my therapist.

So, gentlemen, take cheer! Although the stigma surrounding men's mental health is deeply embedded in societal expectations of masculinity, these stigmas are slowly being dismantled through education, public advocacy, and shifting narratives about what it means to be strong.

We can be part of that change. In fact, you—(yes, you! Right now!)—are part of that change because you're holding this book and taking this journey. Together, we can help create a supportive culture where it's safer to share and easier to heal. That's part of the light at the end of the tunnel I mentioned earlier.

To get to that light, though, we have to go through the darkness. Buckle up, because I'm about to share mine.

COMING TO TERMS WITH THE PAST

Once, while visiting the Florida Everglades, I encountered a tree known as the strangler fig. This deadly fig tree gradually wraps around the trunk of its host, ultimately choking it to death by cutting off access to sunlight, water, and nutrients.

The strangling process begins when a bird or squirrel unknowingly drops a tiny seed near the top of a palm tree. Once the seed finds a nook to germinate in, it sends delicate roots spiraling down the trunk toward the ground. It isn't until these roots reach fertile soil that the strangler fig truly earns its name. Once the roots reach the soil, they thicken and grow, gradually engulfing the tree trunk and starving the host of the vital sunlight it needs to survive.

Ultimately, the strangler fig—known as a hemiepiphyte for those science enthusiasts—kills off the source tree, consuming the decomposing host with its roots.

So why am I talking about trees?

The strangler fig serves as a poignant metaphor for the insidious effects trauma has on our lives. Much like how the fig tree begins as a small seed nestled in the branches of a host tree, trauma often starts as a seemingly insignificant experience, easily dismissed or overlooked. Over time, however, the roots of that trauma grow, winding tightly around our emotional core, much like how the fig tree wraps itself around its host. Slowly but relentlessly, it begins to stifle growth, overshadowing our ability to thrive. What once seemed minor transforms into a force so pervasive it overshadows our capacity to live fully, leaving us ensnared in a web of pain and self-doubt. We may find ourselves struggling to breathe under the weight of past experiences as the vibrant parts of our identity wither away. Like the strangler fig, trauma often takes root without our immediate awareness, leaving us feeling trapped and distant from the light of our true potential.

Let me tell you about my own strangler fig. And to do that, we need to go back to the beginning.

WHERE I CAME FROM

I grew up in a large family in Mesa, Arizona. As the sixth of nine kids, I can safely say I identify as a "middle child." My father, an attorney, had his own real estate litigation practice, and my mother was a stay-at-home mom. I have four brothers and four sisters and countless memories growing up in such a large family. Some of my fondest memories revolve around mealtimes, when we would eat together as a family. In the evenings, my parents would ask how our day went, and if we were lucky, my dad would tell us about the cases he was currently working on. I would especially love it when he would ask us kids for our advice on what he should do to help his clients.

Growing up with loving parents, I knew that one day I wanted to be a good father who not only loved and supported his children but also provided for them and helped them feel safe and secure. Even as a child, I recognized the importance of a strong and cohesive family unit, and I wanted to do everything in my power to provide that for my own family.

Now, a father of three kids, I hope and pray that I'm doing a good job. Having gone through the mental struggles I've faced, there were times when I questioned whether I was truly a good dad. Today, more than eight years after my first panic attack, I can confidently say that I am, in fact, a wonderful dad. I didn't give up, and I certainly didn't give in—and that's what makes me a great dad.

I'll often hear parents say, "I would do anything for my children." Well, I tried to do just that. I threw myself into my healing process knowing that if I wanted to continue to be a good dad, I may have to go to the very depths of hell and back if that is what it took. It just so happens that that's just about what it took to regain my ability to be a happy and healthy father.

When I hear people say, "I would die for my family," I often think to myself, "Yes, that's a noble sentiment, but would you do what it takes to truly *live* for your family? Would you take the necessary steps to *heal* for your family?"

So let's start at the beginning of when my character began to take shape and the events that, for better or for worse, made me the man I am today.

A BOY NAMED WHITNEY

Johnny Cash wrote a song that always brings a smile to my face, "A Boy Named Sue." The song tells the story of a man whose no-good daddy named him Sue before walking out. By the end of the song, Sue explains how grateful he is for his dad and the name he gave him, as it helped him to become a tough man able to survive in a rough world.

Ironically enough, it was also *my* father who named me Whitney. It wasn't to turn me into a fighting, cussing, son-of-a-gun but to remember something important—our pioneer ancestors who settled in the small town of Whitney, Idaho. Granted, Whitney *was* a boy's name for generations, and I found great solace in my early years finding the name "Whitney" under the "Boy's Names" section of baby name books.

Now, before I go into the difficulties of having that name, I want it known that I love my name more than I could ever express.

When I was young, it was hard being a boy named Whitney, but now I wouldn't trade my name for anything in the world. It made me who I am today. Just as Sue thought of his dad, I too credit the majority of my successes and achievements due to the "character building" nature of my name. (So thank you, Mom and Dad, for naming me Whitney. How were you to know it would become a girl's name in the future?) In fact, my name ultimately had such a profoundly positive effect on my life that I even passed it on as my son's middle name.

OK, now back to the story...

In the late eighties, when I was seven years old and trying to make my way through second grade, Whitney Houston burst onto the music scene. Suddenly, my name was on everyone's lips. Instead of basking in the glory of sharing a name with a superstar, though, I found myself the target of relentless teasing. Kids can be cruel, and they seized every opportunity to remind me that I had a "girl's name."

Desperate to escape the constant harassment, I decided the best course of action would be to simply change my name...to Eric. I mean, c'mon, every cool kid I knew in second grade was named Eric. I thought that by shedding the name Whitney, I could finally blend in and find some peace. When I announced my ingenious name-changing plan to my family, they talked me out of it and encouraged me to find a suitable nickname.

Eventually, I settled on going by Whit, hoping that a nickname would offer some relief. But even that wasn't safe from the barbs of my terribly creative classmates. "Nit Whit," "Dim Whit," and "Shit-ney" became their favorite jabs, each one a tiny cut that slowly chipped away at my self-esteem.

As a quiet kid, I often found myself retreating inward, grappling with the constant teasing and the rage it sparked inside me. Internally, I was like a simmering pot, always on the verge of boiling over. I'd clench my fists, grind my teeth, and feel my face flush with anger. At times, I'd lash out verbally, using my quick wit to deliver scathing retorts to my tormentors.

Other times, I would channel my rage into physical outlets, like punching my pillow or a wall, or I'd just zone-out for hours playing *Contra*, *The Legend of Zelda*, or *Super Mario World* on my beloved Nintendo. I remember retreating to our home's basement after school with a large glass of milk and three slices of bread to smooth out my emotions in front of after-school cartoons. This behavior is what probably led to me being a little overweight, as I found "caloric coping" a helpful source of dopamine when I was feeling low due to the day's teasing.

My schoolmates and peers weren't the only ones who teased me. I'll never forget the day my third-grade teacher called me "Nit Whit" in front of the whole class. She'd overhead some of my classmates using the nickname to tease me, and rather than addressing their behavior, she chose to join in.

It was a shocking betrayal from someone I'd trusted and respected. Her tone was condescending and cruel, and the smirk on her face made it clear that she found amusement in my humiliation. It was a moment that shattered my faith in authority figures and reinforced my belief that I was alone in my struggle.

> **"No one can make you feel inferior**
> **without your consent."**
> —ELEANOR ROOSEVELT

FALLING IN LOVE WITH HUMOR

Despite my name being a source of ridicule in my early years, it helped me find (and fall in love with) humor and comedy. At a young age, I fell in love with making people smile, and I believe that's ultimately why I went into dentistry and orthodontics.

When I finally discovered the power of humor, that's when everything changed for me. I figured if I could come up with better jokes about my name than the bullies could, I'd take the wind right out of their sails. I started preemptively striking, armed with an arsenal of self-deprecating quips that left my tormentors deflated and wishing they'd thought of that joke. The humor helped, but it gradually wore on me.

By the time I was eleven, I had very low self-esteem. I felt friendless and alone, desperate for meaningful connections. My parents, doing their best to help me feel loved, believed that spending more time with a male family friend—someone I had once trusted and who was a few years older than me—would help me finally feel like I had a friend. Tragically, unbeknownst to any of us, they were placing me directly into the hands of a predator.

I would spend time with him on the weekends, usually away from our parents. At the time, it was exciting to have someone who was willing to engage with me and make me feel special. Over time, he started to "broaden my horizons," so to speak, by testing my boundaries. It started with lude jokes, then listening to violent and misogynistic music.

We then graduated to mild forms of trespassing and destruction of property. Eventually, he introduced me to risqué movies with swearing and nudity. Whenever I would question whether we should be doing these things, he assured me that "this is how boys become men." He'd frequently ask if I ever told my parents what we did when we were together, and I told him I didn't. I had no desire to break our circle of trust and risk our friendship, so I kept quiet about all of our activities.

It wasn't long after that conversation that he introduced me to pornography, and once again, he reassured me that this was normal behavior for becoming a man. Finally, after he ensured I was keeping our activities secret from my parents and everyone else, he started to sexually abuse me. It lasted for about a year, and I was so ashamed and scared that I couldn't bring myself to tell anyone about it.

I knew on many levels that what he was doing to me was wrong, but I was terrified of losing my connection with someone I mistakenly thought was my friend or being labeled as a pervert. This is when I developed both *toxic shame* and *codependency*—both of which we'll discuss together.

WHAT IS TOXIC SHAME?

Toxic shame[4] is a deeply ingrained feeling of worthlessness or inadequacy, often stemming from negative experiences or criticism in childhood. Unlike healthy guilt, which is linked to specific actions, toxic shame affects your entire sense of self, leading to feelings of unworthiness and self-loathing. It can result in avoidant behaviors, low self-esteem, and difficulties in relationships, causing you to feel unworthy of love or acceptance. Healing from toxic shame often involves therapy and self-compassion to rebuild a positive self-image.

Eventually, I was able to stop spending time with my abuser, but the damage had already been done. If you've ever watched a TV show where someone who's been abused refuses to confide in their parents or authorities and you find yourself shouting at the screen, "Just tell them what happened!"—well, that was me. Overwhelmed by shame and fear, I couldn't tell a soul. I now carried a deep, dark secret that I would hide for years.

I was terrified of my family abandoning me or, even worse, being discovered and labeled as a monster because of my past. This is one of the major effects of abuse. As Jane Middelton-Moz describes in her insightful book *Guilt & Shame: Masters of Disguise*, when a person is abused, especially as a child, they often take on the abuser's shame. For me, this meant blaming myself for what happened—I felt I had allowed myself to be lured, deceived, and taken advantage of.

I tragically convinced myself that it was all my fault, that I was to blame for my abuser's actions. That I had somehow brought this upon myself. Shame has a way of twisting reality, making the victim feel like they deserve what happened to them. I was never the same after that. For years, I held myself accountable for someone else's actions, which only fueled my self-hatred and made me feel worthless.

It's tragic, isn't it? Not only was I hurt through no fault of my own, but I also ended up hating myself for it. Toxic shame can seep deeply into your soul. Sadly, I chose to swallow my pain and fear, burying it deep inside as I tried to move on with my life.

That turned out to be a big mistake, but good luck convincing a scared kid of that.

Eventually, that hidden trauma, guilt, and shame manifested into a multitude of issues that would haunt me later. One of those issues was a deep, burning rage that lingered within me for decades, a process Middelton-Moz discusses in her book.

It wasn't until my time at Sierra Tucson that this pent-up rage was finally released—a story I'll share in Part 4.

> "Shame corrodes the very part of us that
> believes we are capable of change."
> —BRENÉ BROWN

THE PAST IS NOT BEHIND US; IT IS INSIDE OF US

Our past experiences, particularly painful or traumatic ones, can hide deep in our subconscious and sneakily continue to shape how we live, think, and respond to the world. These hidden traumas can manifest in various ways, affecting mental, emotional, and physical well-being. Men, in particular, often struggle to address these traumatic experiences due to societal expectations that discourage emotional vulnerability, making it difficult for them to acknowledge or seek help for their struggles.

A poignant example of how past experiences may be buried deep, hidden from consciousness, came from an unusual story my oldest brother shared with me several years ago. He lived near the beach in Florida, and one day he began experiencing pain in his heel. Initially, he thought it was just a minor discomfort that would go away on its own, but the pain gradually worsened over the course of weeks and eventually months.

Frustrated, he finally visited a podiatrist. After examining the area, the doctor suggested, "I think you may have something lodged in your foot." Though my brother was skeptical, he trusted the doctor's expertise. The podiatrist recommended numbing the area and making a small incision to investigate further.

After numbing the heel with a few injections, the doctor carefully made the incision.

Within moments, he exclaimed, "There it is!"

To my brother's shock, the doctor extracted a large shard of glass. Baffled, my brother asked, "How did that get in there?"

The doctor explained, "It's more common than you think, especially near the beach. People often step on sharp objects in the sand without noticing, especially since there are fewer nerve endings in the heel. Based on the scar tissue, this glass has been in there for quite some time, but it's only now causing you pain."

The glass in my brother's foot is a striking metaphor for the hidden emotional wounds many of us carry—often unnoticed until their painful effects manifest much later.

To help you identify if something harmful or traumatic is embedded in your mind or psyche, I recommend a simple exercise. While sitting in a quiet place, ask yourself this question: "Would I want my child (or future child) to have the same life experiences I had growing up?"

If the answer is yes, consider yourself fortunate—you may not have any embedded "shards" to address. However, if the answer is no, take a moment to write down the painful memories you wouldn't want your child to experience. Reflect on moments when a trusted adult said something hurtful, times you felt betrayed by a friend or loved one, or instances where you witnessed or experienced an accident. Did someone in your life hurt you, knowingly or unknowingly?

As you read this book, keep a pen handy to jot down similar experiences or thoughts. These uncomfortable memories are a signal from your subconscious that something needs attention. Writing them down can be an essential step in the healing process.

When you notice a relevant impression, write it in the margin, dog-ear the page, or note the page number on the front cover if you prefer to keep your pages pristine. If you fall into the "book pages are not to be violated" camp, consider writing your thoughts in a journal instead. Whatever method you choose, I strongly encourage you not to ignore the feelings and thoughts that arise.

These may be buried shards of glass or red flags in your life that desperately need attention before they escalate. Suppressing these emotions can have real consequences— trust me, I found that out the hard way.

> "We raise boys to be 'manly.' They learn to accept pain, never show weakness, and suppress emotions. Then we wonder why men struggle to express their feelings."
>
> -IAIN THOMAS

TYPES OF TRAUMA: THE BURIED SHARDS OF GLASS

There are many forms of trauma that we can experience throughout our lives, and each type has its own sinister way of affecting us. Here's a list to start us off, though it's by no means comprehensive:

- **Childhood Trauma**: Adverse childhood experiences (ACEs) like neglect or abuse can have long-lasting effects into adulthood. Individuals who face trauma may struggle with emotional wounds, such as difficulty forming healthy attachments and fear of abandonment. These early experiences can result in anxiety disorders, attachment issues, or PTSD.[5]

- **Traumatic Loss**: Divorce or the sudden loss of a loved one can lead to intense grief, potentially evolving into complicated grief or depression, often accompanied by guilt that hinders future happiness.

- **Violent Experiences**: Survivors of violence, like veterans or assault victims, may develop PTSD, experiencing flashbacks, nightmares, and hypervigilance, which disrupt daily life and relationships.

- **Chronic Trauma**: Long-term stress from environments like violent neighborhoods or abusive relationships can cause complex PTSD (C-PTSD), resulting in emotional dysregulation and difficulties in forming stable relationships.

The effects of trauma like this can include:

- **Anxiety Disorders**: Past trauma often leads to anxiety, conditioning you to expect danger. For instance, if you were bullied, you may develop social anxiety, fearing judgment in social situations.

- **Depression**: Trauma can instill feelings of worthlessness and hopelessness, especially if you've internalized those negative self-perceptions. This can result in chronic low mood and disinterest in life.

- **Substance Abuse and Addiction**: Unprocessed trauma can drive you to substance use as a coping mechanism, which may lead to addiction and worsened trauma.

- **Physical Health Issues**: Trauma is linked to physical health problems, such as chronic pain and autoimmune disorders, due to stress that weakens the immune system.

Healing is possible through various therapy modalities, such as trauma-focused cognitive behavioral therapy (CBT) and eye movement desensitization and reprocessing (EMDR), which I'll explain more in Part 4. Building support systems is also crucial. Addressing trauma can transform emotional burdens into resilience.

As a result of my shame, I built walls around myself, trapping my emotions deep inside, never letting them see the light of day. I wore a mask, pretending that everything was okay, that nothing had happened to me, and that I was perfectly fine. As the years went on, I pushed further into Whitney the comedian, the clown, always ready with a joke or a witty retort.

I also pushed further into overachievement. I threw myself into every challenge with fierce determination, whether it was academics, sports, or extracurricular activities. I believed that if I could just be the best at everything, if I could accumulate enough accolades and achievements, then perhaps I could finally silence the voices of doubt and derision, both from others and from within myself. I pushed myself to the brink of exhaustion, often sacrificing sleep, social life, and my own well-being in the pursuit of perfection. It was a vicious cycle, as each accomplishment only fueled my need to do more, to be more.

Looking back, I see how using overachievement as a coping mechanism may have helped me succeed in the short term, but it ultimately contributed to my struggles with anxiety, burnout, and a deep-seated sense of never being good enough. It was my way of pushing down the pain, of preventing myself from feeling the full weight of what I'd endured, which only made things worse.

I tried, but ultimately failed, to tell my parents about the abuse. As a frightened child, I didn't have the words to express the full extent of what was happening to me. The guilt, fear, and shame collided into a perfect storm that left me feeling abandoned. It wasn't something I was able to process as a kid, though, and it caught up with me.

But this isn't a story about despair; it's a story about hope. In spite of these traumatic experiences growing up, I didn't give up. I kept going, kept fighting, and believed that one day, I would find a way to heal.

In the end, the trials I faced as a child—whether it was the difficulty of having a girl's name or the burden of being abused— have all been part of making me who I am today. I'm a strong, intelligent, and loving father, husband, brother, and son. Do I wish I could go back in time and change some of my experiences? Of course I do. I believe we all would. But these experiences have all come together to create the recipe that is now Whitney Wright. They've shaped me, but they haven't broken me. They have made me who I am today...and I'm pretty dang awesome if you ask me.

> "Hardships often prepare ordinary
> people for an extraordinary destiny."
> —C.S. LEWIS

MEN UNDER PRESSURE: SPENCER'S STORY

I want to introduce Spencer Caldwell, a childhood friend who endured some difficult traumatic "shards" growing up. Imagine being fourteen years old, hormones raging, your world changing daily. Now add this bombshell: Your parents are divorcing—for the second time.

This was Spencer's reality.

Growing up on a pig farm in Snowflake, Arizona, Spencer's childhood was idyllic until it wasn't. His parents' first divorce when he was twelve was tough, but their second split at fourteen shattered his world.

"The problem with kids when their parents are fighting is that everything feels final," Spencer told me. "When my parents would get in yelling matches and one of them would storm out of the house, I would think, 'I don't know if I'm ever gonna see that person again.'"

On top of the emotional turmoil, Spencer was uprooted from his beloved small town to move to the "big city" of Mesa, Arizona.

As a teen, Spencer found solace in his neighborhood. "I was able to run away from the pain," he shared. A street full of kids became his refuge. Years later, Spencer wrote *Mine Are Too*, a children's guide to divorce. It's the book he wished he'd had as a kid, reassuring young readers that it's not their fault that Mom and Dad are getting divorced. In his own marriage, Spencer made a conscious choice to put family first. "I try to make my spouse number one, be completely unselfish, and be the best father that I can to my kids," he explained.

Spencer's story showcases the power of resilience and perspective. He took a painful childhood experience and transformed it into a tool for helping others.

His journey reminds us that our challenges, however daunting, position us to form our greatest strengths. By facing his past head-on, he healed himself and created a resource that continues to help others.

We have to acknowledge our struggles, learn from them, and then ask, "How can I use this to help someone else?"

In the next chapter, we'll continue to look through that lens—this time, when talking about codependency.

THREE

CODEPENDENCY

T he abuse I experienced as a child made me great at "going along to get along." I didn't want to upset others, so I often avoided conflict and suppressed my own feelings.

Back then, it felt like survival. Looking back today, I can see it was a manifestation of the codependency I developed because of my experiences.

Codependency[6] is a relationship dynamic where one person relies heavily on another person for emotional support, approval, or a sense of self-worth. Often, this involves one person prioritizing the needs and feelings of the other to the point of neglecting their own. The codependent person might feel responsible for the other's happiness or problems, leading to a cycle of dependency where both individuals struggle with boundaries. This can make it hard for them to have healthy, balanced relationships. They may feel trapped in a cycle of giving and sacrificing, while the other person may only take without giving back.

If this sounds familiar, you're not alone. I'm happy to report that now, after extensive therapy, I'm learning to set boundaries and say "no" when necessary. Reflecting on my past, I see moments when I could have stood up for myself, potentially avoiding issues like burnout, depression, and anxiety, but I was too broken inside to take that stand.

Many abuse survivors develop codependent behaviors, often sacrificing their own well-being for the hope of being treated kindly. I often linked my emotions to how others felt about me, prioritizing their happiness over my own. *Psychology Today* defines codependency as a dysfunctional relationship dynamic where one person, "the giver," sacrifices their needs for "the taker."[7] This cycle of "give but then take" creates significant strain on relationships and makes it hard to establish healthy boundaries. I've seen this play out time and time again. In my life, I've faced manipulation and betrayal from a handful of people I trusted, leading to strained relationships and even eventual legal battles, which only exacerbated my mental health struggles. (I recommend *No More Mr. Nice Guy* by Dr. Robert Glover and *Codependent No More* by Melody Beattie for anyone seeking to understand and break free from codependent patterns.)

Breaking free from codependency is challenging but liberating. At Sierra Tucson, I learned to set boundaries and prioritize my own needs. Although it was terrifying at first, as I practiced self-care and allowed others to take responsibility for their emotions, I discovered a newfound sense of freedom and authenticity. True connection, I learned, comes from being whole, not from trying to fill others' voids at the expense of my own well-being.

> **"You don't have to set yourself on fire to keep others warm."**
> —PENNY REID

COPING MECHANISMS

Childhood abuse can leave you feeling invisible. When a child's emotional, physical, and psychological needs go unmet, they may internalize feelings of unworthiness. For me, this created a constant quest for visibility from junior high to college, driven by low self-esteem and toxic shame from my past. My desperate need for validation led me to seek attention through achievements, all while masking deep-seated feelings of inadequacy.

Transitioning from elementary school to junior high was particularly tough. I wanted to be seen, so I ran for student council president in seventh grade and lost. This setback only fueled my determination, and in both eighth and ninth grades, I won. However, each victory felt hollow; my self-worth remained tied to external validation, pushing me to chase more achievements—good grades, laughter as the class clown, and admiration from girlfriends.

This drive for recognition became an addiction, consuming me as I sought to fill an inner void. In high school, I stepped back from student council, embracing the grunge culture of the nineties to rebel against expectations while still yearning for acknowledgment. At times, I engaged in risky behaviors for thrills, masking my rage, which I later realized stemmed from shame.

I focused my energy on my studies, maintaining good grades while cultivating an effortlessly cool persona. In my senior year, I returned to student council and ran for student body president, winning and gaining respect from my peers. I dove into overachievement, believing that accumulating accolades would silence my inner critic.

Looking back, I see how this coping mechanism contributed to my anxiety, burnout, and persistent feelings of inadequacy. In my senior year, I was crowned homecoming king and voted class clown, accolades that provided fleeting validation but ultimately felt empty. Caught in a cycle of seeking approval, I continued chasing achievements, believing they would finally make me feel enough. It wasn't until I'd returned from Sierra Tucson that I finally understood that true worth comes from within, not from external validation.[8]

> "Sometimes, the habits that helped you survive
> will not be the same ones that help you thrive."
> —DR. THEMA BRYANT

TWO VERSIONS OF WHITNEY

Later in life, I would go on to attend Brigham Young University (BYU) and complete a religious mission trip to Argentina—two foundational pieces of my past. While those external mile-stones were shaping my future, though, they couldn't erase the past. Unresolved trauma from my childhood began to bubble up, demanding my attention. I realized that to succeed emo-tionally and academically, I needed professional help.

During my time at BYU, I saw a therapist four or five times to discuss the sexual abuse I'd experienced as a child. While it was a step in the right direction, it barely scratched the surface. Financial constraints as a student made it difficult to continue. Like many abuse victims, I turned to various coping mecha-nisms to numb the shame and anger consuming me. I sadly found solace in pornography, having been introduced to it at a young age by my abuser. I also binged video games like *Halo*, losing myself in virtual worlds. Risk-taking behaviors such as speeding and excessive thrill-seeking became my way of chas-ing a dopamine rush. Without proper treatment, survivors like me are at increased risk for long-term negative outcomes, including higher rates of substance abuse, risky sexual behav-ior, and self-harm.[9]

I risked being one of them. Despite seeking therapy, I strug-gled with a growing sense of duality. I felt like there were two versions of myself: the charming, successful college student everyone saw and the dark, twisted "Evil Whitney" lurking within. I feared that if anyone saw the real me—the broken, angry, ashamed version—they'd reject me.

Breaking free from my painful past proved difficult. The anger and shame felt like a cancer, eating away at me. I con-vinced myself that certain milestones would fix me—serving my mission in Argentina, getting married, having children, graduating from college and dental school. Yet, as each milestone came and went, I found that the healing I craved was always just out of reach. The shame and self-loathing would resurface, no matter how hard I tried to suppress them.

In 2002, I began dating my college sweetheart, Margaret, whom I met in a marine biology class. She said "yes" when I proposed in early 2003. We both graduated from BYU in 2004, and I set my sights on dental school at the University of Colorado, viewing it as the next step in a series of milestones leading to my goal of becoming an orthodontist. I immersed myself in my studies, hoping this new phase would bring the healing I sought. Instead, it introduced new pressures that intensified my internal battles.

Even after marrying Margaret, I relied on my premarital coping mechanisms to keep "Evil Whitney" at bay. I threw myself into my studies and work, attempting to distract myself from the pain. Unfortunately, one coping mechanism in particular only numbed the pain and made me feel worse: pornography. It negatively affected my marriage because I kept this dark secret from my wife.

My abuser had introduced me to it all those years ago, using it to groom and manipulate me. This sickening realization fueled my anger and determination to break free from my past. Getting rid of pornography was at the top of my list for healing. It took years and many slip-ups before I finally stamped out that destructive habit. It wasn't until I was completely honest with Margaret about the depth of my problem that I could free myself. By exposing "Evil Whitney" and admitting my guilt and shame to her, I brought that hidden habit into the light. With her love and support, I finally broke free.

Looking back, I see how destructive that coping mechanism was for my self-worth. Many believe that viewing pornography isn't harmful, but for me, it was a direct link to my abuse. Each time I turned to it to escape my pain, the pain only worsened. I was trapped in a shame cycle, and I knew I needed to break free to move on with my life.

One problem, though: There was more going on underneath the surface.

ADHD, PTSD, AND ADRENAL FATIGUE

When I was a teenager, it felt like I was studying constantly, often sitting at the kitchen table for hours to finish my homework. I often struggled to complete projects and maintain the focus needed for long-term success, reinforcing my toxic shame and belief that I was somehow broken.

Although I'd suspected I had **ADHD**[10] for years, it became clear later in dental school when I couldn't find enough hours in the day to study. While my classmates studied for a couple hours, I'd have to study for four to six hours. Despite always *suspecting* I had ADHD, I hesitated to get tested, fearing it would be seen as a weakness. (Are you seeing a pattern here?) The stigma around ADHD medication loomed large; I grew up believing that needing medication meant you were broken, a perception rooted in the history of Ritalin since its introduction in 1955. This stigma can be a significant barrier to seeking help.[11]

Eventually, I saw a psychologist who confirmed my suspicions—my brain simply didn't function like a neurotypical one. The hyperactivity and impulsivity associated with ADHD fueled my constant need for stimulation and attention, leading me to seek new experiences and achievements to prove my worth. I felt like a failure, blaming myself for my inadequacies.

The disconnect between knowing what I needed to do and actually doing it was incredibly frustrating. It wasn't a matter of apathy; it felt like there was a short circuit between intention and action. I made elaborate to-do lists, only to forget them later. Throughout school, I was cracking jokes while struggling to stay organized. I often forgot assignments and procrastinated, leading to stress and anxiety about falling behind. Living with ADHD was like trying to conduct an orchestra where every instrument was playing a different song at top volume. I joked that I had the attention span of a caffeinated squirrel, bouncing from task to task without completing anything.

At home, ADHD affected my ability to follow through on chores. I'd start tasks with enthusiasm, only to get distracted and leave them unfinished. Socially, my ADHD was both a blessing and a curse. My quick wit made me engaging, but I often struggled with social cues, leading to misunderstandings. I felt like I was working twice as hard just to keep up, which was exhausting.

"You gain strength, courage, and confidence
by every experience in which you really
stop to look fear in the face. You must
do the thing you think you cannot do."
—THEODORE ROOSEVELT

MISUNDERSTANDINGS AROUND MEDICATION

My path to accepting medication for ADHD was not straight-forward; it required confronting deep-seated misconceptions. One of the biggest hurdles was overcoming the stigma associated with medication, which I'd always viewed with skepticism and fear. But seeking help isn't a sign of weakness; it's a step toward unlocking the potential of a unique, brilliant brain.

After years of feeling overwhelmed, I decided to try ADHD medication, and it was transformative. Suddenly, I could focus, sit still, and retain information. It felt like my mind quieted down, allowing me to think clearly for the first time. I remember exclaiming to my wife, "Is this how normal brains work?!"

You might wonder, "Isn't medication just a crutch? Shouldn't you manage ADHD on your own?" ADHD is a legitimate medical condition, not a character flaw. Just as we wouldn't expect someone with diabetes to manage without insulin, we shouldn't expect someone with ADHD to cope without the appropriate treatment.

Armed with the ability to manage my ADHD, I graduated from dental school in 2008 and entered an orthodontics residency at the University of Colorado. For two years, I immersed myself in orthodontics while trying to keep my demons at bay. However, learning to navigate life with ADHD—both with and without medication—revealed a complex paradox: Even with medication, my battle was far from over.

The medical community agrees that identifying and treating ADHD can greatly enhance the physical, mental, and social well-being of those affected. People with ADHD, including myself, often struggle with tasks that others find straightforward, such as interrupting conversations or leaving tasks unfinished. Negative responses from family, teachers, and peers can lead to feelings of inadequacy, complicating their situation further.

This stigma can deter parents from getting their children assessed, causing them to underestimate the risks of untreated ADHD. Delaying diagnosis until adulthood increases the likelihood of early mortality, primarily due to higher risks of suicide and serious accidents due to impulsivity. However, effective treatment can lead to significant improvements in quality of life. And there's good news on the treatment front, including growing interest in nonpharmacological approaches. For more, I strongly recommend the book *Driven to Distraction: Recognizing and Coping with Attention Deficit Disorder from Childhood through Adulthood* by Dr. Edward Hallowell and Dr. John Ratey. Published in 1994, this book brought ADHD to mainstream attention, helping millions understand and manage the condition. I also recommend following that up with their newest book *ADHD 2.0: New Science and Essential Strategies for Thriving with Distraction.*

As I navigated the challenges of living with ADHD, I discovered I wasn't alone. Many others, like those we're about to meet, faced similar struggles, highlighting the importance of recognizing and addressing ADHD—not as a flaw, but as a different way of processing the world.

> **"Your life does not get better by chance; it gets better by change."**
> —JIM ROHN

MEN UNDER PRESSURE: JACOB'S STORY

When Trevor's son Jacob was young, he seemed like a perfect, outgoing kid. He breezed through elementary school with ease, but as he reached junior high, things began to change. His grades slipped from As to Cs—nothing alarming at first, just typical teenage stuff. But this was only the beginning of a challenging journey for both father and son.

In high school, Jacob struggled to read assignments and would complete homework without turning it in. It felt like his brain was working against him, and he could only focus under pressure. One night, while studying for a history test, Jacob described his thoughts: "It's like that huge aquarium at Monterey Bay we visited. All these thoughts are swimming around in circles, and I can't catch hold of any of them."

As his academic struggles mounted, Jacob began experimenting with self-harm and fell into depression. Trevor felt helpless as he watched his bright, funny son fade away. With Trevor's own history of ADHD, he and Jacob's mother decided to have Jacob tested. The results confirmed their suspicions.

"Choosing to get him tested wasn't easy. There's so much stigma around mental health, especially for guys," Trevor explained. Despite this, Trevor and his wife believed it was better to know than to live in ignorance. "Getting that diagnosis was like someone finally handed him the right pair of glasses."

Once Jacob started ADHD medication, his transformation was remarkable. His GPA soared from 2.5 to 3.8. More importantly, Trevor saw his son come back to life, with the happy spark returning to his eyes. "A few months into treatment, Jacob brought me an essay covered in enthusiastic comments from his teacher. He grinned and said, 'I always knew I had good thoughts in my head, but I could never get them out before!'"

Medication wasn't a magic solution, but it leveled the playing field for Jacob. Watching him graduate high school with honors was one of Trevor's proudest moments. Today, Jacob is thriving in college. While ADHD doesn't just disappear, he's learned strategies to manage it and understands that his brain works differently—not better or worse, just differently.

TIME FOR THE BIG LEAGUES

After a grueling ten and a half years of higher education, it was time for me to make my way in the world. Driven not only by the pressure to provide for my family but also by the burden of student loans, I threw myself into my work with reckless abandon. Unfortunately, I still grappled with the demons from my past that thrived on validation, achievement, and accolades. Coupled with my inability to say "no" due to my codependency, this created a perfect storm for failure. The emotional wounds from my childhood—low self-esteem, feelings of worthlessness, and the need to succeed at any cost—pushed me headfirst into the trap of workaholism.

This happened even though I loved my job. Seriously, I *loved* it. From a young age, I dreamed of becoming an orthodontist. I vividly remember my first visit to the orthodontist's office as a shy, self-conscious twelve year old with an overbite and crooked teeth. Watching the orthodontist work his magic captivated me. The fluidity of his office, his precise technical skills, and his ability to transform smiles felt like art in motion.

That moment ignited my obsession with orthodontics. I knew I had to earn top grades to achieve my dream, so I began shadowing my doctor and bombarding him with questions. What I loved most was the combination of art and science, the chance to create beautiful smiles, and the ability to boost others' confidence.

Ultimately, my determination paid off. In August 2008, I was accepted into the University of Colorado Orthodontics

Residency, where I would finally learn the craft that promised fulfillment. However, my desire to become an orthodontist was also about seeking visibility and validation. I won't lie: Part of me craved the thrill of saying, "I am an orthodontist," and the pride that came with reaching that pinnacle.

After graduating in November 2010 and cofounding Risas Dental and Braces with three talented dentists and a savvy business guy, I opened multiple practices but never found the satisfaction I sought, spiraling me right into that other problem: workaholism.

Workaholism is an obsessive preoccupation with work that negatively impacts an individual's personal life, relationships, and overall well-being. It's characterized by an inability to detach from work, often leading to excessive hours spent on job-related tasks, prioritizing work over leisure and social activities, and neglecting self-care. People who are workaholics may feel compelled to work even when it's not necessary and are often driven by a desire for achievement, perfectionism, or fear of failure. This behavior can result in stress, burnout, and health issues over time.

When I think of being a workaholic, I'm reminded of a famous business parable about two men. One, the humble fisherman, knows what his priorities are and protects them well. The other, a workaholic hell-bent on global conquest, can't determine how much success is "enough." It goes like this: An American businessman was vacationing in a small but beautiful beach town in Mexico. While he was drinking his morning coffee on the patio of his hotel, he saw a fisherman coming back to the dock in his small boat and unloading the two large fish he'd caught earlier that morning. After watching the fisherman for several days in a row, the business man approached the fisherman to give him some advice that would surely change his life and put him on a path of success. He asked the fisherman what he does with those two fish every day.

The humble man smiled and said, "I bring them home to my family. We eat the fish together and then spend the rest of the day together laughing and making memories. We do as we please because of the fish that I catch for us."

The businessman was shocked at how small minded this fisherman was. He explained to the ignorant man that if he worked harder, if he caught more fish, if he hired other men to help him catch more fish, he could buy a bigger boat. With a bigger boat, he could hire even more men to catch even more fish and eventually build a fleet of fishing vessels.

The fisherman asked, "And then what?"

The businessman replied excitedly, "Once you have your own fleet, you could buy a large building with lots of expensive canning equipment and machinery and hire hundreds of work-ers. With your own canning operations, you could then begin shipping your canned fish all over the world! You would be rich! Rich beyond your wildest dreams!"

The fisherman smiled and said, "And once I have done all of that, then what do I do?"

The businessman smiled with a far-off look in his eye and said, "Well, that is the beauty of it. Once you've put in all that work, all those years and years toiling to build a fishing and canning empire, that's when you can finally retire and spend your remaining years relaxing. You could get yourself a little boat, catch a couple of fish in the morning, and spend the rest of the day laughing and making memories with your family."

The fisherman knew *how much* was enough for him. He valued time with his family and a simple life in harmony with nature. He didn't need more money, success, or stress to be happy.

That's the lesson I had to learn the hard way, because there's a point at which the pursuit of success becomes self-destructive. We must figure out *how much* is enough, what we truly value, and what we're willing to sacrifice.

Reflecting on the lesson of knowing *how much* is enough, I realized that my pursuit of success had turned my life into a constant juggling act. The wisdom of the humble fisherman struck a chord with me. In my relentless drive for more, I'd lost sight of what truly mattered. I realized that understanding how much is enough wasn't just a simple question—it was a fundamental shift in how I approached my life and work.

Sadly, the trauma of my early years had a way of compounding over time. Just as the strangler fig chokes out its host, my former traumas made me feel like I was dying on the inside. I didn't realize it then, but the coping mechanisms I developed to deal with the shame and hurt—the overachievement, the people-pleasing, the workaholism—were setting me up for a massive reckoning later in life. Little did I know that the very things I thought would set me free—the accolades, the achievements, the relentless pursuit of success—would ultimately bring me to my knees.

"He who knows that enough is
enough will always have enough."
—LAO TZU

PTSD ENTERS THE PICTURE

Years later, Risas Dental and Braces was thriving, and my wife and I had several children. Yet I often felt like I was constantly trying to fill a bucket riddled with holes—which ultimately left me feeling drained and unable to feel truly alive. Mentally and emotionally, I was in a tough spot. Balancing the demands of my practice—seeing over one hundred patients a day—while trying to be a present father, a supportive husband, and an active leader in my congregation felt overwhelming. I could relate to Bilbo Baggins in *The Fellowship of the Ring* when he said, "I feel thin, sort of stretched, like butter scraped over too much bread."[12]

I was wearing too many hats and felt busier than a one-legged man in a butt-kicking contest...only to realize I was kicking my own butt. Although I'd learned to manage my ADHD, an unsettling emotion lingered—anger. This simmering presence needed to be confronted before it consumed me entirely.

As I navigated the challenges of dental school and cofounding my practice, I began to experience a deep, inexplicable anger that felt like a fire in my belly, threatening to engulf me. I later learned this inner turmoil is common among those who have faced trauma. Research indicates that childhood trauma can increase anger and aggression in adulthood[13] and raise the risk of mental health issues like PTSD and depression.[14]

I realized I'd bottled up my anger for years, pretending it wasn't there. Like a shaken soda can, the pressure was building, and it was only a matter of time before it exploded. One incident stands out: A colleague made an offhand comment suggesting I didn't deserve to be an orthodontist and hadn't contributed meaningfully to the company—that I cofounded! This comment triggered deep-seated feelings of inadequacy. I'd worked hard and sacrificed much for my education and our business, and their implication that I was unworthy reinforced traumas tied to feeling invisible—what's known as "imposter syndrome," which is characterized by self-doubt and inadequacy despite evident success.[15]

Suddenly, all the rage, pain, and hurt I'd been suppressing surged to the surface, and I felt on the brink of exploding. While I didn't become violent, my words dripped with venom and spite, cutting deeply. I don't think my colleague intended any harm, but in that moment, it felt like an attack on my very identity, a reminder of all the times I'd felt invisible and unworthy of love and respect.

This incident served as a wake-up call, revealing that I couldn't keep running from my past or pretending everything was okay. Pain demands to be felt, and no matter how hard I tried to escape it, it always caught up with me. This echoes the words of trauma expert Bessel van der Kolk, who stated, "The body keeps the score."[16] Unresolved trauma can manifest as physical symptoms and emotional dysregulation long after the initial event. The anger, shame, and trauma within me were building to a breaking point, and I finally admitted that

I couldn't continue living this way. I needed help—fast. I didn't realize at the time that I was struggling with **PTSD**.[17]

> **"PTSD is not the person refusing**
> **to let go of the past, but the past**
> **refusing to let go of the person."**
> —DR. JUDITH HERMAN

FEELING LIKE A STRANGER IN YOUR OWN LIFE

PTSD can arise after someone experiences or witnesses a traumatic event, such as an accident or violent incident. Those with PTSD may relive the trauma through flashbacks or nightmares, feel constantly on edge, or struggle with sleep. They might avoid situations that remind them of the trauma, making daily life overwhelming. Essentially, PTSD is your mind's way of grappling with a painful experience, hindering your ability to feel safe and move forward.

My carefully constructed façade began to crumble as the reality of my PTSD emerged. This was more than just stress or burnout; it was deep, unresolved trauma that influenced my every action. Like many who have faced trauma, I learned that the symptoms can sneak up on you and turn your life upside down.

PTSD is akin to living with a hair-trigger alarm system in your brain, going off at the slightest provocation. A car backfiring, an unexpected touch, or even a particular smell can transport you back to the trauma, heart racing and palms sweating, primed for fight or flight. This constant state of high alert is exhausting.

One of the most frustrating aspects of PTSD is feeling like a stranger in your own life. Things that once brought joy become sources of anxiety. Relationships suffer because you're unable to relax or be present. The trauma creates a before and after in your life, leaving you mourning the person you used to be while struggling to navigate a new hypervigilant reality.

After World War I, returning soldiers faced similar challenges, experiencing flashbacks, insomnia, and withdrawal. Many turned to alcohol or other vices to numb their feelings. The medical community eventually recognized that the horrors they witnessed altered their brains, dubbing it "shell shock." As time passed, similar symptoms emerged in victims of car accidents or abuse. PTSD can arise from any traumatic experience that disrupts your mental well-being. It wasn't until the 1980s that PTSD was officially recognized as a diagnosis, highlighting its far-reaching impact.

The body doesn't lie about trauma-PTSD affects several parts of the brain. The hippocampus, which helps with memory, is often smaller in people with PTSD.[18] The amygdala, which controls emotions, tends to be more active, making fear responses stronger.[19] At the same time, the prefrontal cortex, which helps with decision-making and emotional control, may be less active, making it harder to handle stress and emotions.

Essentially, living with PTSD means your body remains in fight-or-flight mode, never being able to fully calm down or relax. I didn't know that I had PTSD until it stopped me in my tracks.

And it wasn't the only thing that kept me stuck there.

HELLO, ADRENAL FATIGUE

After years of pushing myself to the brink in my orthodontic offices while burying my pain and anger, I started shutting down mentally and physically. Feeling like a walking zombie with no energy or zest for life, I chalked it up to stress from building a business and being a new dad. But when my energy plummeted and I had severe brain fog, I knew something was wrong.

I talked to one of my brothers, who reported that he'd just discovered he had low testosterone. So, with a renewed determination to start feeling better, I scheduled an appointment with my general physician to talk about getting tested. I finally made it to the appointment, hopeful that I'd feel better soon.

I told the doctor about my low mood, lack of energy, and mental fog. I told him my brother just tested critically low on testosterone and that I'd like to be tested. What happened next, I'll never forget. The doctor looked at my arms and said, "You have hair on your arms; you're just fine. There's no need to test your testosterone."

I was shocked at his flippant dismissal of my concerns and his unwillingness to just order a simple blood test! My hopes of feeling better were dropping, and fast. I went home upset and confused, and I told my wife what had happened. Luckily, she suggested I find another doctor to get checked. I'm so glad I did. It turns out that you can have plenty of hair on your arms and still have very low testosterone. I never went back to that doctor again.

While trying to understand what was happening to my body while living with undiagnosed PTSD, I uncovered another hidden battle: adrenal fatigue. The relentless stress and pressure had pushed my body to its limits, and the effects were undeniable. I remember visiting a naturopathic doctor who ran a battery of tests to check over a hundred different factors in my blood, from testosterone levels to kidney and liver function. After discussing my symptoms, my breakneck pace at work, and the various challenges I was facing, he suggested even further tests. He believed I was suffering from more than just low testosterone; I was experiencing full-blown adrenal dysfunction, commonly known as adrenal fatigue. The adrenal glands, small organs located on top of each kidney, are responsible for producing adrenaline and cortisol. When he tested my adrenal levels and the amount of neurotransmitters my brain was producing, the results were concerning—everything was extremely low, leading to his diagnosis of **adrenal fatigue**.[20]

Adrenal fatigue is a condition where the adrenal glands become overworked and less efficient at producing hormones like cortisol, which help regulate stress. Many believe this occurs after prolonged periods of stress, resulting in exhaustion, sleep disturbances, and a general lack of energy. Symptoms can include fatigue, difficulty concentrating, and cravings for salty or sweet foods. While it's not officially recognized as a medical diagnosis, many people feel their bodies struggle to cope with daily stresses, leading to a sense of burnout.

What I didn't realize at the time was that my body was in a constant state of fight or flight due to the PTSD. This response is fueled by adrenaline, one of the adrenal glands' primary functions. With my adrenal glands working overtime to keep me going, it was like running an engine at high RPMs all the time—eventually, something has to give. Just as someone who consumes too much sugar and ignores their doctor's medical advice can develop type 2 diabetes due to pancreatic burnout, my adrenal glands also became depleted.

That's exactly what happened to me. I burned out, both physically and mentally. It wasn't until I was later diagnosed with PTSD at Sierra Tucson—a condition I'd always associated with soldiers returning from war—that it started to make sense why I had burned out. However, trauma comes in many forms, and the battles I faced in my personal and professional life left their mark.

MEN UNDER PRESSURE: BRIAN'S STORY

In the world of business and personal development, we often encounter stories of triumph over adversity. However, few narratives capture the essence of resilience quite like the journey of my friend Brian. His story serves as a powerful illustration of how unexpected life events can test our limits and ultimately reshape our approach to both personal and professional challenges.

I've known Brian since our junior high days. A skilled mechanic and devoted family man, he's the craftsman behind Clementine, my prized orange 1973 K5 Chevy Blazer. His expertise in restoring dilapidated vehicles would soon be put to the test in rebuilding his own life after a devastating family crisis.

On an ordinary Arizona afternoon, Brian's world was upended when his teenage son was involved in a severe motorcycle accident. Despite wearing a helmet, he collided with a cinder block wall at high speed. By sheer fortune, a quick-thinking homeowner performed CPR, bringing Brian's son back from the brink of death.

Brian's son endured intensive medical intervention for a traumatic brain injury, including hours of surgery and extensive facial reconstruction. The psychological impact of these events was profound, manifesting in Brian as adrenal fatigue and depression, slowly eroding his typically resilient demeanor. This strain extended to his marriage, as differing approaches to their son's care created a rift between Brian and his wife. Additionally, the mounting medical bills and rehabilitation costs added significant financial pressure, compounding the already tense situation and making it even more challenging for the family to navigate their ordeal. Sadly, Brian's marriage fell apart under the weight of blame and resentment, leading to a significant strain on his mental health that affected his work and relationships. The family dynamic was forever altered, and they had to completely restructure their lives as they struggled to adapt to the new reality brought on by the accident.

Despite overwhelming challenges, Brian demonstrated remarkable resilience. He took the crucial step of seeking professional help for his adrenal fatigue and depression, understanding the importance of addressing his mental health. Adopting a methodical approach to recovery, Brian focused on small, achievable goals, taking it day by day. He leaned on his support network to navigate the emotional turbulence, recognizing the value of having a strong support system. Additionally, Brian developed new coping mechanisms and adjusted his expectations for the future, adapting to the new realities of his life with determination and strength.

Brian's story serves as a powerful reminder that life can change in an instant, but it's our response to these changes that ultimately defines us. Throughout our lives, we're often faced with unexpected challenges that test our limits. His journey demonstrates that with perseverance, support, and the right mindset, we can not only weather the storm but emerge stronger on the other side.

The next time you're facing a seemingly insurmountable obstacle, remember Brian. Remember that even in the darkest times, there's always potential for growth and renewal. It may not be easy, it certainly won't be comfortable, but with grit and determination, you can navigate any tempest your life or business throws your way.

"Chronic stress is a silent killer. Listen to your body before it's too late."
—DR. MARK HYMAN

BATTLING ADRENAL FATIGUE

Adrenal fatigue is like trying to run a marathon on fumes. Your body's stress response system is so overworked and depleted that even the smallest tasks feel Herculean. I remember days when just getting out of bed felt like scaling a mountain. My energy levels were so low that I needed a nap after taking a shower. Feeling utterly drained all the time was frustrating and demoralizing.

While "adrenal fatigue" isn't a recognized medical diagnosis, the symptoms people describe are very real. It can feel like your whole body is rewired, especially your stress response system. Research from Psycotherapy Today shows how long-term anxiety keeps the hypothalamic-pituitary-adrenal (HPA) axis stuck in overdrive.[21] When your brain is constantly signaling danger, your adrenal glands keep pumping out stress hormones like cortisol. At first, this might help you stay alert, but over time, it wears you down. Your body starts struggling to regulate hormones, your immune system takes a hit, and you're left feeling drained, foggy, and more prone to illness. It's like revving an engine nonstop—you can only go so long before something gives out.

It's also true that chronic stress pushes the adrenal glands into overproduction at first but eventually burns them out, according to the Institute for Functional Medicine.[22] That's when you hit full-on exhaustion mode—low energy, brain fog, trouble handling stress, and even hormonal imbalances. And it's not just about feeling tired. According to data published in the Society of Behavorial Medicine, long-term stress messes with more than just your mood—it triggers inflammation, metabolic problems, and even increases the risk of serious diseases.[23] In other words, this isn't just in your head. Adrenal fatigue can be a full-body experience—and if left unchecked, it can take a serious toll on your health.

I know because I've been there. Adrenal fatigue can sneak up on you. We live in a culture that glorifies busyness, pushing ourselves to the brink in the name of productivity. I wore my exhaustion like a badge of honor, convinced that pushing just a little harder would lead to a breakthrough. Instead, I crashed spectacularly—a harsh wake-up call that our bodies have limits, and ignoring those limits comes at a steep cost.

Recovering from adrenal fatigue is a slow process that requires a complete lifestyle overhaul. (There's good news: It's amazing how powerful practices like meditation can be in restoring balance to our overworked systems.) Understanding my own adrenal fatigue has given me insight into the struggles others face and has helped me better understand myself—including the fact that I was also facing anxiety and depression.

DEPRESSION AND ANXIETY

t this point in the story, I was a complete mess! Here I was, an ADHD codependent workaholic dealing with unresolved trauma, battling undiagnosed PTSD, and fighting adrenal fatigue. It was safe to say I was "tore up from the floor up." But does the list end there? Nope. I'm not sure when the **depression**[24] and **anxiety**[25] started to creep into my life, but thankfully my therapist caught it and sent me to a psychiatrist to get some much needed help.

Depression is more than just feeling sad; it's a complex mental health condition that affects how you think, feel, and handle daily activities. Imagine a heavy cloud hanging over you that makes everything seem dull and difficult, even things you used to enjoy. People with depression often experience persistent feelings of hopelessness, fatigue, and worthlessness, which can make it hard to get out of bed or concentrate on tasks. It's not a sign of weakness or something you can just "snap out of." Depression can change your brain chemistry and may be triggered by a variety of factors, including genetics, life events, or chemical imbalances. The good news is that it's a treatable condition, and with the right support—like therapy, medication, or lifestyle changes— many people can find relief and start to feel better.

Depression is a sneaky beast. It usually doesn't announce itself with dramatic sadness or tears. For me, depression crept in like a thick fog, slowly dulling the colors of my world until everything felt flat and gray. I'd find myself staring at the wall for hours, feeling nothing but a vast emptiness where my emotions used to be. It was like being trapped behind a pane of glass, able to watch but unable to fully participate in life.

The COVID-19 pandemic really threw a spotlight on the prevalence of depression. A 2023 meta-analysis in *The Lancet* showed that rates of major depressive disorder increased by a whopping 28 percent globally in 2020. That's millions of people suddenly grappling with the black dog of depression, often without access to their usual support systems.

Depression is the most common mental health disorder among middle-aged men. Unlike women, men often experience and express depression differently, with symptoms such as irritability, anger, fatigue, and physical complaints like headaches or digestive issues being more prevalent. In addition to depression, anxiety disorders and substance use disorders are also commonly seen in this demographic.[26]

Tragically, middle-aged men (ages forty-five to sixty-four) have the highest suicide rate among all age groups in the United States, with a rate of approximately 30.6 per 100,000 individuals. This rate is significantly higher than the national average across all age groups, highlighting the severe mental health challenges men in this demographic face.[27]

Luckily, my psychiatrist prescribed me some medication to help pull me out of the doom-spiral of depression. It took a few tweaks to get the dosage correct, but once it was right...I once again started feeling Wright!

> "That's the thing about depression: A human being can survive almost anything as long as they see the end in sight. But depression is so insidious, and it compounds daily, that it's impossible to ever see the end."
>
> —ELIZABETH WURTZEL

ANXIETY: ANOTHER KICK IN THE TEETH

Anxiety is like having an alarm system in your body that goes off too often, even when there's no real danger. It can leave you feeling constantly on edge, worried, or restless, as if you're anticipating something bad to happen. People with anxiety might experience racing thoughts, a pounding heart, or even physical symptoms like sweating or shaking. Everyday situations—like speaking in public, meeting new people, or just going to work—can feel overwhelming. It's crucial to understand that anxiety isn't merely feeling nervous; it can significantly disrupt daily life and relationships. The good news is that effective treatments, such as therapy and medication, can help individuals manage their anxiety and regain control.

One of the most insidious aspects of anxiety is how it can masquerade as productivity. I often found myself consumed by worries about all sorts of possible, often catastrophic, scenarios. I told myself it was just my Eagle Scout training—"being prepared" for what might come next. In reality, I was trapped in a muddy rut of what-ifs and worst-case scenarios. It wasn't until I learned to recognize and challenge these anxious thoughts that I realized how much mental energy I'd been wasting.

When anxiety peaks, your brain perceives danger, triggering the fight-or-flight response and flooding your bloodstream with adrenaline. This creates a positive feedback loop: The adrenaline heightens your anxiety, which prompts even more adrenaline, and so on. This terrifying cycle can spiral until your body can't take it anymore. In my case, the emergency response my body chose was a panic attack instead of a heart attack. A panic attack occurs when your brain and body become so overwhelmed with anxiety that they attempt to release that pent-up energy in a desperate bid to keep you alive. For me, this manifested as hyperventilation, profuse sweating, and often ended with me vomiting and crying uncontrollably on the floor. Tragically, my body learned to cope with anxiety through panic attacks, and it would default to this response every time my anxiety spiked. It's absolutely terrifying and humiliating to lose control of your mind and body in this way. Even writing this brings tears to my eyes as I recount the pain and fear involved. When I mentioned at the beginning of the book that my main motivation for sharing my story was to prevent others from experiencing what I've gone through, this is precisely what I meant.

The physical manifestation of anxiety isn't something I'm alone in experiencing...far from it. It's well documented that we often feel anxiety in our bodies as well as our minds—and that those physical manifestations can be harmful to our health. For example, research shows that having an anxiety disorder increases your risk of developing cardiovascular disease, and if you already have heart issues, you're more likely to develop anxiety. It's a loop that can be hard to break without targeted intervention. And it's not just the worry itself—anxiety affects sleep, encourages unhealthy coping mechanisms (like smoking or overeating), and makes exercise feel like an insurmountable task, all of which contribute to declining heart health.[28]

And then there's the long-term impact of anxiety, especially for people who have experienced chronic stress or early-life trauma. Research has shown that people with a history of adverse childhood experiences were more likely to develop both anxiety and heart rhythm issues later in life. Their study suggests that unresolved anxiety from past trauma can linger in the body, slowly chipping away at cardiovascular resilience. It's not just about what's happening right now—your anxiety could be carrying the weight of past stressors that continue to impact your physical health.[29]

On a brighter note, research is uncovering new ways to tackle anxiety. A 2022 study in *Psychological Medicine* found that the way your brain processes stress and emotions before therapy might influence how much it helps, which could lead to more personalized anxiety treatments in the future.[30] This potential to tailor treatment plans based on our unique brain wiring gives me hope for more individualized, effective approaches to managing anxiety in the future—but for now, we've got to work with what we have and keep pushing forward.

> **"If you're going through hell, keep going."**
> —WINSTON CHURCHILL

LOOKING AHEAD

The good news is that neither depression nor anxiety is untreatable. The techniques I learned at Sierra Tucson for managing my disorders were transformative. Meditation and breathwork became my go-to strategies for grounding myself when panic threatened to bubble up, for instance. We'll unpack these strategies together more in Part 4. For now, let's consider what happens when all these challenges combine, stewing in your brain and making you feel like you're spiraling out of control. Can you picture what likely happened next?

You guessed it: one first-class ticket to burnout, please.

BURNOUT AND BREAKDOWN

t was now 2016, five years into starting Risas Dental and Braces. I was on various medications—Wellbutrin for depression, testosterone for low levels, adrenal fatigue supplements, and a daily Xanax to manage my anxiety. Yet I couldn't stop pushing myself to the brink of exhaustion, trapped in a cycle of seeking validation through overworking. I was addicted to the high of achievement, always chasing the next big win, unable to slow down, take a break, or recharge. Enter *burnout*.

Burnout[31] is a state of physical, emotional, and mental exhaustion caused by prolonged stress, often from work or demanding responsibilities. Imagine feeling completely drained, like your battery is running on empty, and no matter how much you try to recharge, you just can't seem to regain your energy. It's more than just being tired; it can make you feel cynical, disengaged, and hopeless about your tasks. You might struggle to concentrate, lose interest in things you once enjoyed, or feel overwhelmed by even simple tasks. Essentially, burnout happens when you push yourself too hard for too long without giving yourself the care and time you need to recover.

I ignored the red flags: panic attacks, physical and emotional exhaustion, and constant overwhelm. I convinced myself I was invincible, but that wasn't true. Eventually, when I had to transition to solely doing managerial work—because I experienced panic attacks every time I sat in the orthodontist chair, even while working on my own kid's braces—I realized I'd been running on empty for so long that I had nothing left to give. It felt like driving a car at full throttle for years without changing the oil or checking the tires, inevitably leading to a breakdown. I was in burnout...but I kept pushing. I couldn't stop.

MEN UNDER PRESSURE: MICHAEL'S STORY

When I first heard Michael Levitt speak at an orthodontic convention about his book *Burnout Proof*, it was like looking into a funhouse mirror of my own life. Here was a guy who'd nose-dived into the abyss of burnout and somehow clawed his way back out. His story hit me like a root canal without anesthesia—painful, but boy, did it wake me up.

Michael had been your typical overachiever, burning the candle at both ends and probably in the middle, too. But unlike some of us who manage to catch ourselves before we go over the cliff, Michael's story took a swan dive into the deep end of burnout. You might be wondering how a seemingly successful person can end up in such a mess. In his book, Michael outlines a laundry list of reasons that contribute to burnout, including people-pleasing, a lack of boundaries, poor diet, insufficient exercise, inadequate sleep, low self-confidence, past traumas, workplace issues, feeling out of control, isolation, social media addiction, and a mismatch between your values and your job or relationships. Each of these factors can create a perfect storm, pushing us to our limits.

In May 2009, at the ripe old age of forty, Michael had a heart attack. Now, I've had some rough days in my life, but I can't imagine anything scarier than feeling your own ticker betray you when you're barely into your fourth decade. For Michael, this wasn't rock bottom—the universe had more in store for him.

"In one year, I had a heart attack that should have killed me. I also lost my job during an economic recession, the family vehicle was repossessed, and then finally our home was foreclosed," Michael told us, his voice a mix of disbelief and hard-won wisdom.

It was like the guy was living through a country song, minus the part about the dog running away.

But here's where Michael's story takes a turn for the awesome. Instead of letting this tsunami of crap drown him, he decided to swim. He started making changes—big and small—anything to get his life back on track. He ensured he got seven to eight hours of quality sleep each night by maintaining a consistent sleep schedule and a relaxing bedtime routine. To keep work from encroaching on personal time, he set clear boundaries, designating specific hours for work and personal activities to ensure he had time to recharge. By tracking expenses, setting financial goals, and avoiding unnecessary spending, he reduced his financial stress and gained greater control over his life.

Michael regularly decluttered his living and working spaces, creating an organized and calming environment that reduced stress and enhanced focus. Daily journaling allowed him to reflect, process experiences, set intentions, and stay grounded and self-aware. He focused on high-impact activities, eliminated nonessential commitments, and delegated tasks when possible to maximize productivity and minimize stress.

The result? Michael didn't just recover; he reinvented himself. He then wrote *Burnout Proof*, sharing his hard-won wisdom with others. Now he travels around, speaking at conferences (like the one where I met him), helping other people avoid the burnout cliff he tumbled off.

Michael's story is a wake-up call, but it's also a beacon of hope. It shows that even when you've hit rock bottom—when you've lost your health, your job, and your home—you can still turn things around. It's not easy, and it's not quick, but it's possible.

As I sat there listening to Michael speak, I couldn't help but feel a mix of emotions. There was relief—knowing I wasn't alone in my struggles, that other successful people had faced similar demons. But there was also a challenge. If Michael could bounce back from such a catastrophic burnout, what was stopping me from making changes in my own life?

Michael's journey from burnout to breakthrough isn't just inspiring—it's a roadmap for anyone who's feeling overwhelmed, stressed, or on the verge of burning out. It's a reminder that small changes can lead to big results and that it's never too late to turn your life around.

So the next time you're feeling like you're running on empty, remember Michael's story. Take a step back, reassess your priorities, and don't be afraid to make big changes. Your health—physical, mental, and financial—depends on it. And who knows? Maybe one day you'll be the one standing on a stage, sharing your own story of transformation. Stranger things have happened.

"The cure for burnout isn't rest. It's finding something to love that energizes you."
—GREG MCKEOWN

PUSHING PAST THE RED FLAGS

My workaholism wasn't sustainable, but it took time—and a series of red flags—for me to see that. I ignored the warning signs for far too long, convinced that if I just worked harder, everything would be okay.

After starting medication for depression, anxiety, and adrenal fatigue, I thought things would improve. I believed I could finally breathe and focus on growing the company sustainably. However, the pressure to overwork myself remained. When I voiced my concerns to a mentor, he said, "When I feel down, I just work harder. I get more productive. That's how I push through it." At the time, that seemed like sound advice. I thought that by working even harder, I could ignore the red flags around me. So I did just that, pushing myself to the brink of exhaustion and burnout. I felt that if I wasn't constantly expanding and growing the company, I wasn't good for anything.

Just before the panic attacks started, I remember one day driving to my fourteenth office in just five years, crying behind the wheel, feeling like I was heading into a dumpster fire that was waiting to ignite. I felt like I was drowning under the weight of expectations and responsibilities. When I arrived at work, I had to sit in the car for a few minutes to compose myself, put on my "Dr. Wright" persona, and pretend everything was okay. That day, I saw 115 patients, joking and laughing as usual. But it was all a façade. Inside, I was falling apart. Maintaining that façade became increasingly difficult as the months wore on. I was running on empty, burning the candle at both ends. I knew I was headed for a crash, but I felt I had no choice but to push on.

Looking back, I can see how foolish and reckless I was. I was risking my health and well-being for a misguided sense of duty. So focused on being the hero, I neglected to take care of myself. But hindsight is 20/20. At the time, I was just trying to survive, convinced that if I could make it through one more day, everything would be okay. Of course, everything was not okay. Things were about to get a lot worse before they got better.

As our company continued to grow, I found myself in a cycle of starting new practices only to leave them behind once they were up and running. This bittersweet experience took a heavy toll on my mental health and was one of the leading contributors to my PTSD. In each new office, I felt like the king of the castle. I'd blast eighties tunes, sing along, and keep everyone laughing with my endless jokes. I loved the energy and excitement of building something new and creating a welcoming space for patients.

However, each new practice also meant saying goodbye to patients I had poured my heart and soul into. It felt like breaking up with someone you loved, over and over again. I felt like I was letting people down, abandoning them when they needed me most. Over five years, I said goodbye to more than seven thousand patients across fourteen practices—a staggering number that weighed heavily on my heart.

When I would revisit those offices, the patients would let me know in a roundabout way that I'd disappointed them, saying, "I wanted you, Dr. Wright, to do my braces, but you left me," or "I like my new orthodontist, but he isn't you." Each time, it felt like a gut punch. How could I leave behind all those patients who trusted me? Sadly, I eventually stopped visiting those offices; it became too painful to be there.

I felt trapped. My job was to start new practices and hire doctors to take them over, but the constant cycle of hello and goodbye was destroying me from the inside out. I later discovered that this recurring trauma would lead to another aspect of my already thriving PTSD: I was chronically reliving the trauma of each goodbye every time I walked into a new office. I'd lie awake at night, my mind racing with the faces of patients I'd left behind, wondering if they felt abandoned and alone.

This burden grew heavier with each passing year. Despite my efforts to push through, I knew I was reaching my breaking point.

> "The cost of a thing is the amount of life
> which is required to be exchanged for it."
> —HENRY DAVID THOREAU

DEVASTATING PANIC ATTACKS

When the panic attacks finally hit, it was unlike anything I'd ever experienced. It felt like being overwhelmed by a tidal wave of fear and anxiety with no escape. I remember the first time clearly: It was a particularly stressful day at work, juggling countless tasks. I was working on a patient, and then all of a sudden I fell out of my chair and onto the floor. I stood back up dazed and fell against the wall to my left. Suddenly, my chest tightened, my heart raced, I broke into a full-body sweat, my vision blurred, and I couldn't catch my breath. I thought for sure I was having a stroke.

I tried all my usual coping mechanisms—deep breathing, positive self-talk, visualization—but nothing worked. I felt like a kite caught in a hurricane, completely at the mercy of the storm. As the panic attack progressed, my anxiety intensified, creating a vicious cycle of fear and dread. I shook uncontrollably, my stomach churned, and my eyes burned with tears. The adrenaline surged, and I thought my heart might explode. I rushed into the restroom, where I collapsed onto the floor, a puddle of sweat, tears, and vomit, utterly drained of every ounce of energy.

This level of hopelessness was new to me. I felt like I'd lost control of my body and mind, like a prisoner in my own skin. The panic attacks grew more frequent until I could expect to have one every day I was seeing patients. The fear of losing my career kept me from discussing it openly, but after a particularly bad episode, I knew I couldn't continue like this. I finally told my business partner (that savvy business guy) Jeff Adams, the CEO of Risas, that I needed a break to rest and recover. He was genuinely worried about me and agreed that I needed to step back, even though I didn't like the idea because I felt like I was letting the team down.

I felt I had betrayed myself, failing to meet the impossible standards I had set. I was supposed to be Dr. Whitney Wright, the invincible orthodontist, but here I was, broken and defeated.

After a lengthy conversation with my business partner at the end of 2016, we decided I would stop practicing orthodontics and focus solely on the managerial side of the business. This decision resulted in a significant pay cut, but it was the only way to prevent self-destruction. I will forever be grateful for his kindness and understanding during such a terrifying time in my life. Honestly, I truly mean it when I say I love that man like a brother.

And just like that, my career as an orthodontist was over. After only five years in a profession I loved, I was burned out, broken, and utterly lost. The career I'd worked so hard to achieve, the countless hours of studying despite my ADHD, and the fears I'd faced throughout my schooling—all of it felt in vain. I'd spent my life striving to become an orthodontist, and now I was forced to stop because of my own hubris.

How difficult is it to become an orthodontist? First off, you have to be at or near the top of your dental class and have incredible entrance exam results and stellar letters of recommendation, not an easy feat when dealing with ADHD. To help put it into perspective, in the US, according to the American Dental Association, 6,500 dentists graduate annually.[32] And according to the American Association of Orthodontics, only 390 orthodontists graduate each year—meaning only 6 percent of dentists are able to become orthodontists.[33]

Looking back, I see how I reached that point: I'd pushed myself past my limits, ignoring warning signs and red flags. I sacrificed my well-being for a misguided sense of duty and responsibility. At the time, I didn't know any other way to be.

I'd always been a high achiever who could handle anything. I thought if I kept pushing, grinding, and hustling, I would eventually come out on top.

But that's not how it works. There's only so much the human body and mind can take before they break down. No amount of willpower or determination can fix that once it happens. It was a hard lesson, but one I needed to learn. As painful as those panic attacks were, they ultimately served as a wake-up call, prompting me to reevaluate my priorities and finally put myself first.

The panic attacks and the loss of my career woke me up to the fact that I'd been living my life all wrong. Despite the pain, I'm grateful for those experiences. They taught me valuable lessons about boundaries, self-care, and the importance of prioritizing myself. While I may never go back to the way things were, I know I'm stronger, wiser, and more resilient because of what I've been through. I now have the tools and knowledge to build a fulfilling life that aligns with my deepest values and desires.

If there's one thing I want you to take away from my story, it's this: Don't wait until you're broken to start figuring out what truly matters. Don't push yourself past your limits in pursuit of external goals or validation. Take the time to know yourself—understand your needs, wants, and values. Set boundaries and stick to them, even when it's hard or uncomfortable.

Because at the end of the day, life is about the relationships we build, the experiences we have, and the memories we make. If we prioritize these things and our well-being, we can create a truly rich and fulfilling life, no matter the challenges.

"Our anxiety does not empty
tomorrow of its sorrows, but only
empties today of its strengths."
—CHARLES SPURGEON

THE FINAL BREAKDOWN

The final breaking point came to a head in the beginning of 2019 during what should have been a routine director's meeting. Instead, it became the moment that everything I'd been trying to hold together finally fell apart. We were discussing expanding into Texas and opening a new office in Chandler, Arizona.

A good portion of the Texas expansion was my responsibility, as I needed to recruit and train the doctors who would be going there. We also had no orthodontists lined up for the Chandler office, which was opening very soon, so one of the directors innocently asked me if I was feeling healthy enough after taking three years off from practicing to reprise my role as the clinical orthodontist and start seeing those patients again until we could find a suitable replacement. I instantly felt a massive wave of emotions come crashing down on top of me. It was a mixture of a deep sense of loss, mourning the fact that I was no longer working hands-on with patients, and severe dread and anxiety at the thought of returning to the clinic. I started spiraling.

Over the last couple of years, the responsibility of recruiting and onboarding new dentists to staff our new offices had been taking its toll on me. The pressure of feeling as though the overall success of a new office depended entirely on my ability to find the best candidates weighed on me like a ton of bricks. Suddenly, in the middle of the meeting, after two years of no panic attacks, I felt the tightness in my chest, racing heart, and full-body sweat signaling a panic attack. This one was different—more intense than anything I had ever experienced.

I stumbled out of the meeting room and headed for the bathroom, my vision tunneling and breath coming in short gasps. I could hear my colleagues' concerned voices calling after me as I made my way down the hall, but I couldn't focus on anything except the overwhelming fear and dread consuming me.

My colleagues knew I had struggled with anxiety and burnout, but they thought it was in the past. They had only seen the happy, smiling Dr. Wright who handled everything with a joke and a grin. In that moment, they saw me for who I really was—a man barely holding himself together. Luckily, my friend and colleague Jase recognized what was happening. He followed me into the bathroom to lend his support. After the attack subsided, he helped me escape out the back door to my car and stayed with me until I felt okay to drive home. His comfort and support were unforgettable.

Driving away, I knew something had to change yet again. I couldn't keep pushing myself to the brink of a breakdown. That final panic attack was a clear signal that I needed help, and I needed it now. When I got home that day, I told my wife what had happened. Sobbing, I confessed how sad and defeated I felt, knowing the panic attacks had returned despite all the progress I thought I'd made.

The panic attack was devastating, but it was also a turning point. It forced me to take a step back and seek help, leading me to Sierra Tucson, where I would begin to rebuild my life.

THE PATH TO HEALING

The next day, I saw my psychiatrist, hoping for answers. Instead, she told me I needed to stop working immediately and check into a thirty-day treatment facility for anxiety, depression, and burnout. If I didn't, she would stop seeing me as a patient, concerned my panic attacks would escalate into something worse.

I was devastated. Leaving my family and responsibilities for a month felt impossible. But my incredibly wonderful wife supported me, agreeing with the doctor and encouraging me to do whatever it took to get better. The hardest part was telling my kids. While on a weekend getaway, I broke the news, explaining why Dad needed to go away for a while. Their confused, fearful looks were heart-wrenching, as they worried *they* had done something wrong, that maybe Dad was broken beyond repair.

I felt it, too—the sense of brokenness, of being an empty husk. I knew I needed help, but admitting it was terrifying. But I did it. I packed my bags and checked into Sierra Tucson, a treatment facility in Southern Arizona for all types of clientele, from the recovering drug addict to the high achievers who have pushed themselves too far.

Admitting the need for help was the bravest thing I could do—it allowed me to rediscover myself and reconnect with my family. For so long, I lived on autopilot, chasing the next achievement, accolade, or external marker of success. I thought if I worked hard enough, I could outrun my pain and prove I was invincible. But no one is invincible. We all have limits, breaking points, and moments of vulnerability. There's no shame in that. In fact, these moments often reveal our greatest strength and resilience.

If you're struggling with your own unseen battles, know this: You are not alone. You are not broken or weak for needing help. It takes tremendous strength and resilience to face our demons and confront the parts of ourselves we've kept hidden.

"The only way out is through."
—ROBERT FROST

WHAT'S NEXT?

In Part 2, we'll explore strategies to consider if you're struggling. With determination and commitment, these actions can serve as a foundation for healing, helping you approach life's burdens with renewed confidence and resilience. Why? Because I think you and I can both agree that "keeping on keeping on" only works for so long, and we're worth the effort.

PART TWO

WADING INTO THE WATERS

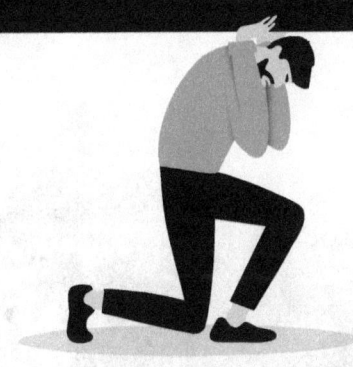

SEVEN

A FOCUS ON THE MIND AND BODY

ong before my final panic attack and eventual check-in at Sierra Tucson, I started making course corrections in my life in an attempt to feel better. At the time, I didn't realize I was grappling with hidden issues that were preventing me from truly healing, no matter how hard I tried. What I did know was that something had to change, and I made the decision to take action to reverse the downward spiral.

When someone isn't feeling their best, one of the first pieces of advice from experts is to incorporate exercise and improve their diet. This often includes cutting back on alcohol, tobacco, drugs, and sugary foods or drinks. Exercise doesn't have to be intense—something as simple as getting outside for a walk is a great starting point, with the eventual goal of reaching thirty minutes every day.

Having dabbled in weightlifting as a teenager, I was familiar with the basics, but after fifteen years of leading a sedentary lifestyle, I realized I needed guidance. In 2014, I signed up to work with a personal trainer at the local gym, and it turned out to be one of the best decisions I ever made. Beyond the physical benefits, there were emotional rewards as well. My trainer, Kris, pushed me to go beyond what I thought were my limits, helping me not only improve my health but also build confidence in myself.

To my surprise and delight, I discovered that "Kris" was short for Kristen. After months of working out together, I jokingly asked him, "Hey, Kris, when are we going to talk about the fact that we both have girl names?" He froze, looked at me in horror, and asked, "How did you find that out?!" As it turned out, Kris's name reflected his Irish heritage, much like how my name, Whitney, was a nod to my ancestral town of Whitney, Idaho. This shared experience over our unique names created an instant bond. Having both grown up navigating the challenges of our names, we found an unexpected common ground.

I trained with Kris three times a week for many years. On our very first day, he asked me about my fitness goals. I kept it simple and said, "I want to be able to do a pull-up." With a confident smile, he replied, "You'll do more than one." That promise set the tone for our training and the supportive camaraderie that followed.

Surprisingly, instead of diving straight into pull-ups, we started with flexibility exercises, light weightlifting, and cardio. Kris insisted I trust the process, emphasizing the importance of building a strong foundation. After about four months, Kris finally announced, "Today is pull-up day!" I felt a wave of panic—pull-ups had always been my nemesis. I imagined myself awkwardly dangling from the bar in front of the entire gym, futilely attempting to lift my six-foot-two, 235-pound frame.

Kris, however, was confident and reassured me I was ready. To my absolute shock, I managed to crank out seven pull-ups! Kris cheered and laughed the entire time, clapping and celebrating my unexpected strength. That moment was a game-changer. The sense of accomplishment was electrifying, and from that day on, I was hooked on the gym, fueled by the desire to see what other limits I could break.

Over time, Kris and I shifted our focus to all-around fitness, emphasizing foundational lifts like barbell squats, deadlifts, and bench presses. Thanks to his careful coaching and guidance, my strength steadily increased year after year. I'll never forget one particularly intense week when Kris challenged me to test my maximum potential in the three major lifts.

With each session, we progressively added weight to my barbell workouts, and by the end of the week, I achieved personal records: 345 lbs on the squat, 385 lbs on the deadlift, and 280 lbs on the bench press. Kris broke into a wide grin and said, "Welcome to the thousand-pound club!" Confused, I asked what he meant. He explained that the thousand-pound club is an unofficial milestone for lifters who can cumulatively lift 1,000 lbs across those three exercises.

I was stunned—and deeply grateful to Kris for guiding me to such a monumental achievement, a goal I hadn't even known existed. He had a knack for pushing me beyond what I believed was possible, from those first pull-ups to joining the thousand-pound club. His belief in me made all the difference.

Kris became more than just a trainer—he became one of my closest friends. The beauty of a friendship built on mutual support is that you both rise together. As a natural leader, Kris eventually became the manager of one of the largest gyms in Arizona, showcasing his ability to inspire and guide others.

In 2020, Kris transitioned careers, embarking on a new journey as a financial advisor after completing a rigorous series of courses. Fortunately, before leaving the fitness industry, he asked me to be his workout partner. To this day, we still hit the gym together four to five times a week, keeping the routine alive.

Kris remains one of my best friends, and having someone to regularly talk to and confide in has been essential to my well-being. His friendship has proven to be just as impactful as his guidance in the gym, reminding me of the power of connection and support in every aspect of life.

So just get moving. Start small, get your blood flowing, and see how much better you feel.

MEN UNDER PRESSURE: ALAN'S STORY

As I sat across from my friend Alan, observing him fidget with nervous energy in the early afternoon, I marveled at the journey that had led him to discuss his mental health with me. At forty-five, Alan is a father of six, a devoted husband, and until recently, a business owner. However, he also battles anxiety and insomnia, often cycling himself into exhaustion. It's a life story he never imagined for himself, but as I've learned through my own exploration of mental health, life has a way of throwing unexpected curveballs.

Alan's story is not unique; millions grapple with anxiety daily. Yet his coping mechanisms are a bit more intense than your average meditation app. "To cope with my anxiety, I go out on my road bike and try to absolutely exhaust myself, pushing my body to its limits," Alan explained, his eyes lighting up with a mix of desperation and determination. But before diving into his two-wheeled therapy sessions, let's rewind a bit.

The year 2020 hit Alan's life like a freight train, and his business was right in its path. "During the COVID shutdowns, month after month, we were losing tens of thousands of dollars," he recounted, the stress evident in his voice. "By November, we were asking ourselves, what do we do? The state was threatening another shutdown." On top of this, his father's battle with Alzheimer's—"the longest funeral ever," as Alan grimly joked—added to the constant pressure of not failing his family, creating a perfect cocktail for anxiety.

"I can't fail my wife or kids," he stated, his voice tight with emotion. "I have this huge responsibility on my shoulders. My family has been my primary concern since the day I got married."

So how do you cope with this storm of stressors? Apparently, by creating a morning routine that would make most people question their sanity. "I wake up at 3:45 a.m., roll out of bed, make a preworkout drink, journal, read some scriptures, meditate, say prayers, and then I get dressed and ride my bike."

I was both impressed and concerned by the intensity of Alan's routine. But as he explained each element, I began to see the method in his madness. Journaling helps him process the chaos of the previous day. Scripture and prayer connect him to something larger than himself. And the bike? Well, that's where the magic happens.

It turns out there's something beautifully simple about cycling, Alan told me. It's just him, the bike, and the open road—no room for anxiety when you're focused on avoiding becoming roadkill at 5:00 a.m. But for Alan, cycling serves as a metaphor for life itself. Sometimes he's cruising downhill with the wind in his hair; other times, he's grinding up steep inclines, every pedal stroke a battle. Yet he keeps going because that's what he does.

"I like to keep my cards close to my chest," Alan explained, a mischievous glint in his eye. "At local races, I show up in jeans and a T-shirt, and people think I'm a goofball. Then I surprise them by beating them. I love that." It's not just about the physical exertion (though by the end of a fifty-mile ride, his legs are screaming louder than his anxiety ever could). It's about proving to himself, day after day, that he can do hard things, face his demons, push through the pain, and emerge stronger.

Of course, no rider makes it through the Tour de France alone. His wife—whom he speaks of with unmistakable adoration—has become his unofficial therapist. "I did one thing right in my life: I married my wife," he told me with palpable sincerity. His faith, too, provides perspective, reminding him that this life is just one leg of a much longer journey. "I am so grateful for my religion because I don't know where I'd be without it. It's been an anchor for me," he shared.

So where does all of this leave Alan? Still anxious, still waking up at obscenely early hours, still pedaling as if his life depends on it (because in a way, it does). But he's also stronger, more resilient, and proud of the miles he's covered. To prevent his body from succumbing to the stress of his rigorous miles and early wake-up calls, Alan embraces the principle of "early to bed, early to rise," usually going to bed around 8:00 p.m.

His business? They ended up selling it—a plot twist Alan never saw coming. But like an unexpected detour on a long ride, it has opened up new paths he never knew existed. His family remains his north star, the reason he keeps pushing forward even when every fiber of his being wants to quit.

And Alan himself? He's still that unassuming guy on a bike, surprising everyone (including himself) with what he's capable of. Because that's the thing about anxiety—it whispers that you're weak, that you can't handle what life throws at you. But every morning, as Alan clips into his pedals and pushes off into the darkness, he proves it wrong.

I'm struck by the unique and powerful way Alan has found to manage his anxiety. While his methods may be extreme, they emphasize the importance of finding personalized coping strategies that resonate deeply. Alan's story reminds us that the path to mental health is as individual as the person navigating it—whether walking or cycling.

"Success is the sum of small efforts repeated day in and day out—this applies to both diet and exercise."
—ROBERT COLLIER

DAILY GROUNDING HABITS

Taking care of our physical bodies is one part of the healing process; another is taking care of our minds. One of the things I started doing to avoid sinking deeper into depression, for example, was giving my mind a break from the stress of my busy work life. With ADHD, my mental gears are always turning. When I face a problem, I can fixate on it, relentlessly focusing on solving it. The issue is that my mind often fixates on multiple problems simultaneously, leading to feeling overwhelmed as I try to juggle several tasks at once. It's like being a dog with multiple bones, unsure of which one to tackle first and instead feeling paralyzed by indecision. Relaxing my mind becomes crucial when I start spiraling out of control.

Meditation is one of the most effective ways I've found to calm my thoughts. When I first tried meditation, I thought it was more complex than it is. But I eventually learned it's as simple as controlling your breath and focusing on that one task.

Try it with me now: Breathe in through your nose for four seconds, counting them in your head. Then breathe out through your mouth for four seconds, counting again. Keep repeating this process, focusing solely on your breathing, and soon you'll find yourself meditating. If your mind starts to wander, which it inevitably will, don't get frustrated. Imagine your thoughts as a puppy learning to stay in its bed. When the puppy strays, you wouldn't scold it; you'd gently guide it back. Do the same with your wandering thoughts—gently bring them back and refocus on your breathing.

Another excellent form of meditation is guided meditation, which many apps can help with. One of my favorites is Insight Timer, and I highly recommend the guided meditations by Sarah Blondin. Her voice and approach are pure gold, offering a soothing path to relaxation. Along with meditation, daily journaling has been a game-changer for me. It doesn't have to be lengthy or profound. Even keeping a simple gratitude journal can work wonders in fending off negative thoughts.

Writing down three things you're grateful for each day shifts your mindset from one of feeling like a victim to recognizing your victories. You're winning at life more than you might realize. A gratitude journal can help you see how well things are actually going.

Lastly, prayer has been a grounding practice that centers me. It doesn't matter who or what your higher power is—just talk to them. Whether you pray in the morning or at night before bed, this practice brings a sense of security. For me, that higher power is God, and knowing that He has a plan for me has helped alleviate much of my anxiety and depression.

When your thoughts feel overwhelming or if you're feeling lost, take a moment to breathe, reflect on what you're grateful for, and give thanks to your higher power for those blessings. You'll likely find a sense of calm and clarity emerging.

MEN UNDER PRESSURE: TANNER'S STORY

Just as anxiety shaped my life, I discovered that others, like Tanner, faced similar challenges in different contexts. Tanner, a man who appeared to have it all, was quietly wrestling with the debilitating anxiety I knew all too well. His story illustrates that anxiety doesn't discriminate; it affects everyone, regardless of outward success.

I first met Tanner in high school, but it wasn't until we reconnected professionally years later that I truly got to know the man behind the suit. A force of nature in the business world, he juggles multiple ventures with the finesse of a seasoned circus performer. However, as I learned, even the most composed professionals have their breaking points.

Picture this: Tanner, the epitome of the successful businessman, always impeccably dressed in his shirt and tie (even during the COVID-19 quarantine!), facing the usual stressors of running multiple businesses while navigating the heart-wrenching journey of parenting a child with a congenital heart defect.

"I always thought that pit in my gut was my X factor," Tanner confided one day. "When things get really stressful and challenging, it's like I just take on more." Sound familiar? It's that classic overachiever mindset many of us fall into—we think we're invincible until we aren't.

For him, the breaking point came when he was blindsided by a panic attack. "I might as well have been physically vomiting. I can't describe it any other way. It was like complete emotional nausea," he recalled, still tinged with disbelief at the memory.

Here's where Tanner's story takes an inspiring turn. Rather than trying to power through or dismiss it as a onetime event, he chose to confront the storm head-on. The solutions he devised are as impressive as his business acumen:

- **The Morning Routine**: Tanner implemented a rigorous morning routine that would impress even the most disciplined individuals. This includes meditation, prayer, exercise, gratitude practice, and reading—all before most of us have even hit the snooze button. "Those five things, no matter what, I try to do every morning," Tanner explained. He doesn't just do it; he feels like he *has to* do it.

- **Hot Yoga**: As someone who tends to run hotter than a furnace, I had my reservations about this one, but it works wonders for Tanner! "I can reach a deep state of relaxation that I've never experienced in regular yoga," he shared.

- **Weekly "Realignment" Sessions**: Think of it as taking your car in for a tune-up, except the vehicle is your life, and the mechanic is...well, you. Tanner described it this way: "Just like your tires need to be balanced or realigned, we need to do the same in our lives. If we keep driving without stopping, that's when we get a blowout. I sit down and write a personal inventory of how my life is going well and where it isn't. I make suggestions to myself as if I were counseling a friend. If I would tell my friend to bail on a situation, that's what I tell myself, too. It helps me stay focused on the best aspects of my life and let go of the worst."

The impact of these changes on Tanner's life has been nothing short of transformative. He's now managing stress and anxiety better, handling personal and professional challenges with newfound grace, and—most importantly—he's found a sense of balance and perspective that once felt impossible.

Perhaps the most powerful outcome has been Tanner's openness and vulnerability. "Honestly, Whitney, when you told me about your panic attacks and your struggles with anxiety and depression, it blew my mind. Your honesty was a gut punch and served as a wake-up call for me to slow down," he admitted.

He later shared that parenting a child with a heart defect requiring multiple surgeries and, ultimately, a transplant in her teens is an ongoing challenge that demands constant presence and adaptation. However, he's learned to focus on the present rather than constantly worrying about the future. "I've tried to enjoy today and be present because I don't know what tomorrow brings," he said.

I want to leave you with one final thought from Tanner: "Nobody's going to care about my life as much as I should." It's a powerful reminder that while support from others is crucial, the real work of maintaining balance and mental health starts with you.

So, to all you overachievers out there pushing yourselves to the limit, remember Tanner's journey. Take a breath, realign, and have the courage to face your own storms. You might just discover, as Tanner did, that there's calm and clarity waiting for you on the other side.

EIGHT

A FOCUS ON FINANCES

One of the best decisions my wife and I made (mostly thanks to her) was to focus on managing our finances and work toward becoming completely debt-free. When I graduated from my orthodontic residency in 2010, I'd spent over ten years in higher education and was now staring down more than $475,000 in student debt that grew every day. My lifelong budgeting approach had been simple: If there was money in my bank account, I could buy whatever I wanted. Unsurprisingly, this led to some difficult conversations between my wife and me over the years, especially since she was the one trying to balance our accounts and make everything work.

I've always dreaded budgeting. It makes me feel trapped and constrained. If there's one thing I loathe in life, it's feeling trapped; it ranks right up there with feeling manipulated.

So, with much difficulty on my part, we decided to align our goals and tackle our finances using Dave Ramsey's *Total Money Makeover* process. As he famously says, "If you live like no one else, later you can live like no one else." After reading his book, we became "gazelle intense," tracking every dollar and employing the snowball technique to pay down our loans one at a time. We chose to focus on the smallest loans first to build momentum.

As we began to chip away at each loan, we created a Loan Board—a large piece of construction paper where we listed all our loans, the payments we'd made, and how many were left. It felt incredible to make multiple payments each month and watch our debts shrink. Eventually, we paid off all our student loans and car loans.

Finally, all that was left was our mortgage. We debated heavily on whether or not to pay off our house since the loan had such a low interest rate.

The turning point came after enduring several lawsuits related to the company—cases we ultimately won, but at a significant cost. The constant legal battles left my wife and me feeling threatened, disrupting our peace and happiness. Seeking a greater sense of security amid the ongoing litigation, we decided it was time to become completely debt-free. After consulting my dad, who had paid off his home following the recession of the late eighties, he advised, "I don't know anyone who has ever regretted paying off their house." Given his background as a real estate litigation attorney, his words carried weight, so we decided to pay off the house.

So we leaned even further into our budgeting and finances to pay off our final loan. I'll always remember the day we wrote that final check to the bank. My dad was right; it felt incredible to know that our home was completely ours and that nobody could take it away from us. I realized that if everything fell apart—if I lost my job or became unable to practice orthodontics—we would still have our home. Little did we know just how prophetic that would turn out to be.

> "A big part of financial freedom is having your heart and mind free from worry about the what-ifs of life."
> —SUZE ORMAN

MEN UNDER PRESSURE: BECKETT'S STORY

At twenty-four, Beckett felt ready to conquer the world as he began working for his father-in-law's fence company. However, he was unaware that he was about to embark on a tumultuous journey marked by depression, financial turmoil, and marital strife, before ultimately finding his path to recovery and redemption. Hailing from Southern Colorado, Beckett married young at twenty-one and quickly ventured into entrepreneurship by launching his first fence business. After that venture failed, he joined his father-in-law's established fencing company, where he managed a team of twenty-five people. Over the next several years, Beckett faced numerous challenges that threatened to overwhelm him, including severe depression and anxiety, significant weight gain peaking at 270 pounds, and mounting financial debt. He also dealt with marital difficulties and career instability, leading to frequent job changes and addictive behaviors related to social media and alcohol use. Feeling increasingly disconnected from his children, he recalled, "I spiraled really deep into depression, relying on Zoloft and other weight-gaining antidepressants and anti-anxiety medications."

The 2008 economic crisis forced Beckett to transition to the oil fields. While this move was initially challenging, it eventually led to better financial opportunities. Later, he even started his own fence installation business. A pivotal moment came in 2017 when he discovered some financial advice that clicked. "I called my wife and said, 'I think we should try this debt snowball thing.' And she replied, 'Yeah, I've been telling you that forever!'"

One immediate benefit was the near-total elimination of his debt. Years of financial mismanagement had taken a toll, but with renewed focus, he tackled his financial issues head-on. They went all-in on getting out of debt and taking full control of their financial lives. By setting up a disciplined budget, cutting unnecessary expenses, and negotiating with creditors, Beckett gradually reduced, then fully eliminated, his debt. The sense of relief that came with achieving financial stability was indescribable, allowing him to concentrate on other vital areas of his life.

Professionally, Beckett's efforts bore fruit in the form of a thriving nationwide fence installation business. With the mental clarity and determination gained from his recovery journey, he scaled his business beyond his wildest dreams. By implementing new strategies, building a strong team, and focusing on excellent customer service, his business is now a source of pride and purpose.

Beckett's transformation also revitalized his marriage and strengthened his bonds with his children and family. His emotional and mental well-being allowed him to reconnect with loved ones on a deeper level. Additionally, he experienced dramatic weight loss and improved physical health, enhancing his overall quality of life. His journey even led him to reconcile with his estranged brother, mending a long-standing source of pain. He admitted one of the biggest factors in his healing was reconnecting with his faith and rekindling his relationship with God. These collective outcomes contributed to an enhanced outlook on life and a profound sense of fulfillment.

Beckett's journey to redemption is a powerful testament to the human capacity for change and growth. Through persistent effort, support from loved ones, and a willingness to face his challenges, he transformed his life. He encapsulates the essence of his transformation: "You've got to do different things, reprogram your brain to accept new information, and take it in a whole different direction."

Beckett's story serves as an inspiring example of what can happen when you get your financial house in order. Whether you do that by going all-in on reducing your debt, making your first budget, or opening a savings account, the point is that you do *something*. That you start. I am here to tell you: There's tremendous stress relief on the other side of the money-trouble mountain.

NINE

A FOCUS ON HONEST COMMUNICATION

One of the side effects of being a victim of abuse is the tendency to become a people pleaser, which is often referred to as codependency (as we discussed in Chapter 3). Those who have suffered at the hands of someone in authority learn early on that it's better to go along to get along. Unfortunately, I was no different. People pleasers often exhibit several key tendencies that can significantly impact their mental health and relationships. Here are some common traits and behaviors associated with people-pleasing:[34]

1. **Difficulty Saying No**: People pleasers struggle to decline requests, even when they don't want to take something on, leading to overcommitment and eventual resentment.

2. **Extreme Anxiety Around Others' Feelings**: They tend to feel anxious when they think someone's upset with them, often going out of their way to rectify the situation.

3. **Taking Responsibility for Others' Emotions**: A strong tendency to assume that others' feelings are their responsibility can lead to guilt or distress if someone else is unhappy.

4. **Conflict Avoidance**: People pleasers often go to great lengths to avoid disagreements, fearing negative reactions or judgment from others. This avoidance can result in built-up tension and frustration.

5. **Need for External Validation**: Many derive their self-worth from the approval of others, perpetuating a cycle of seeking validation and neglecting their own needs.

6. **Perfectionism**: They may strive for perfection in their efforts to please others, fearing that any flaw might lead to rejection or abandonment.

7. **Hyper-vigilance**: Constantly monitoring other people's moods and reactions can lead to anxiety and a feeling of being on edge, as people pleasers seek to ensure everyone around them is happy.

8. **Burnout**: The stress of trying to meet everyone's needs can lead to emotional and physical exhaustion, as people pleasers often prioritize others over their own well-being.

Sadly, one way I exhibited many of these traits was by not honestly communicating with my wife. Because of my codependent behaviors, I often withheld my true feelings and desires, sacrificing my own wants to be what I thought was "a good husband." Ultimately, this led to arguments about how at times I didn't feel loved in our relationship. I felt it was sometimes one-sided—that I was putting in more effort to make her happy than she was to make me happy. These built-up resentments and frustrations created an unhealthy dynamic in what was otherwise a loving relationship. A pivotal book that helped me realize the damage my dishonesty was causing is *No More Mr. Nice Guy* by Dr. Robert Glover, which completely transformed how I viewed my relationship with my wife and others. His book helped me realize that our relationship was not one-sided, but my destructive codependent tendencies blinded me to all the things she was doing to show her love and appreciation to me, all the time.

Once I committed to improving my communication and becoming a more whole person, I discovered *His Needs, Her Needs: Building a Marriage That Lasts* by Dr. Willard F. Harley, Jr. This book includes exercises at the end of each chapter for asking and answering questions with your partner, which were an absolute breakthrough for me. Even after twenty years of marriage, I learned so much about my wife, and she learned about me in return. (Men, can you fully explain the difference between affection and intimacy and how the balance of those two crucial things play a massive role in your relationship? If not, get Harley's book. You're welcome.) Another insightful read on the importance of honest communication is Jordan B. Peterson's *12 Rules for Life: An Antidote for Chaos*. This book helped me realize that by being honest and authentic at all times—no matter what—I would ultimately come out on top. It also reinforced that striving to be a virtuous man is one of the highest ideals.

By finally being honest with myself and others, I found my stress levels decreasing, my heart feeling lighter, and my interactions becoming more authentic. Gone are the days of going along to get along. If something doesn't work for me or my family, I'm going to speak up—sorry, but not sorry.

> **"Honesty and transparency make you vulnerable. Be honest and transparent anyway."**
> —MOTHER TERESA

MEN UNDER PRESSURE: KEVIN'S STORY

As I watched Kevin, a bona fide people pleaser, adjust his tucked-in shirt for the umpteenth time, fussing over his reflection in the office window, I couldn't help but see a bit of myself in his nervous dance. He was about to step into a significant meeting with his boss, and the tension radiating off him was palpable. But this wasn't just garden-variety nerves—no, this was the look of a man preparing to don a mask so seamless, so practiced, that even he might forget it wasn't his true face.

"You've got this, Kev," I offered, trying to inject some reassurance into his pregame ritual. He flashed a smile that didn't quite reach his eyes, and I knew he was already slipping into character—Perfect Employee Kevin, reporting for duty.

Codependency is a sneaky beast, transforming you into a chameleon desperately trying to blend in with whatever environment you find yourself in. And Kevin? He was the poster child for this shape-shifting act.

I've witnessed my fair share of trauma and dysfunction, but Kevin's story was different. He grew up in a pressure-cooker home with a military dad who ran the family like basic training and a mom obsessed with keeping up appearances. Talk about a recipe for people-pleasing perfection.

"My old man," Kevin once confided, his voice tight, "had two modes—disappointed and not-yet-disappointed. I became a frickin' expert at tap-dancing my way into that second category."

That tap dance became Kevin's whole life. At work, at home, with friends—he was constantly scanning, adjusting, morphing into whatever he thought others wanted him to be. It was exhausting to watch him, let alone live it. He would do anything to keep his father from erupting into one of his fits of violent rage that often ended in bruises and blood.

"I don't even know who I am anymore," he admitted during one of our late-night chats. "It's like I'm this hollow shell, and I just pour in whatever personality is needed for the moment."

Sound familiar? I thought it might. We all have a bit of that chameleon in us, but for Kevin, it had consumed his entire existence—and it took a toll. The storm truly broke for Kevin when his marriage began to crumble. Turns out, being a human mood ring isn't great for intimacy. Who knew? His wife called him out for never having an opinion, for always deferring to her desires. Poor Kev was so accustomed to shape-shifting that he couldn't even articulate what he wanted. It was like watching a computer crash in real-time. All those years of suppressing his true self and bending over backward to please everyone else—it all came crashing down. In the rubble, Kevin finally had to confront a painful truth: He had no idea who he really was.

I'm no stranger to facing your demons, but witnessing Kevin start to unpeel his layers of false selves was something else entirely. He started small—saying "no" to overtime when he didn't want to work late, expressing a preference for Chinese over Italian when asked about dinner plans. Baby steps, but for Kevin, they were monumental.

"It feels like I'm learning to walk again," he told me, a mix of excitement and terror in his voice. "Every time I express a real opinion, I feel like I'm waiting for the other shoe to drop, for someone to call me out as a fraud or, even worse, physically hit me."

And here's the beautiful thing: The sky didn't fall. The world didn't end because Kevin said he preferred action movies over rom-coms. Slowly, albeit painfully, he started to uncover the real Kevin beneath all those masks.

It wasn't all sunshine and rainbows. There were plenty of stumbles along the way. Old habits die hard, and Kevin's people-pleasing instincts were deeply ingrained. But with therapy, a lot of self-reflection, and a metric ton of patience, he began to make real progress.

The Kevin I see now? He's still a work in progress (aren't we all?), but there's an authenticity to him that's downright refreshing. He laughs easier, argues when he disagrees, and—get this—actually knows what he wants most of the time.

"I feel like I'm finally living my own life," he told me recently, a genuine smile lighting up his face. "It's scary as hell sometimes, but it's mine."

In the end, we all desire the courage to be ourselves, warts and all, in a world that often seems to demand perfection. Kevin's journey from codependency to authenticity is a reminder that it's never too late to start being real.

So the next time you find yourself reaching for that familiar chameleon's mask, take a page from Kevin's book. Pause. Take a breath. And ask yourself: "What do I really want? Who am I beneath all these roles I play?" The answer might surprise you—and trust me, it's worth discovering.

A great book I can recommend for anyone wanting to learn what is truly good for you in your life at this moment, and how to say "NO" to all the other things, is *Essentialism* by Greg McKeown. It is a fantastic read for just about everyone!

As for Kevin? He's still adjusting his shirt as he heads into that big meeting. But this time, the face reflected in the window is all him. And let me tell you, authenticity looks good on him.

A FOCUS ON SETTING BOUNDARIES

ooking back on my journey, there are many things I wish I'd done differently. I learned countless lessons the hard way, through trial, error, and a great deal of pain. One of the most significant lessons was the importance of setting boundaries to protect myself. If I had established clear limits and articulated my needs without fear of repercussions, my career and life might have turned out differently.

Soon after returning home from Sierra Tucson, I found a therapist who combined traditional therapy with yoga. Intrigued by the approach, I scheduled an appointment. Our sessions took place in my home, and at first, everything seemed to be going well. One of our primary focuses was my deep frustration with others manipulating and taking advantage of me. We worked on recognizing these patterns in my life and setting boundaries to protect myself.

Little did I know just how soon I would need to use those very strategies—against him.

One day, after a session ended, he casually mentioned that he was going through a financial rough patch and asked if I could prepay for a few sessions to help him out. His request felt a little off, but I wanted to be supportive, so I agreed. After all, I believed in helping people when I could.

Then, the next day, I received a text that sent me into a complete tailspin.

"Whitney, I hate to ask this of you, but I've been struggling to find more work, and I have several bills due soon. I hate to ask this, but can I have a loan to keep my affairs in order? I'll pay you back as soon as I'm able."

I couldn't believe it. Here was the very person I'd confided in about my struggles with being taken advantage of—and he's now trying to do exactly that! It was a complete violation of my trust and our professional relationship.

A flood of emotions—anger, betrayal, disbelief—washed over me. But once I calmed down, I knew exactly what I needed to do. I'd spent too much time learning how to set boundaries to ignore this red flag. So I responded with firm clarity:

"I'm very sorry you're facing these financial challenges. However, your request has irreparably changed our professional relationship. Please keep the money I prepaid for our next sessions as a gift to help you during this time. That said, I am officially ending our sessions together."

The old codependent version of me—the one who hated disappointing people—probably would have caved, offering the loan even though it made me uncomfortable. But I wasn't that person anymore. I was a new man, determined to take care of myself. So I fired him.

He sent multiple apology texts, trying to smooth things over and regain my trust. But the damage was done. I held firm to my boundary and never responded.

This time, I chose myself. And that choice made all the difference.

Setting boundaries is essential for maintaining mental and emotional well-being. Boundaries help define personal limits and protect our physical and emotional space, allowing us to cultivate healthier relationships. By clearly communicating what we are comfortable with, we reduce the risk of burnout and resentment, especially for individuals who tend to be people pleasers or codependent. Research shows that setting boundaries is linked to increased self-esteem and reduced anxiety, as it empowers individuals to prioritize their own needs. Furthermore, establishing boundaries encourages respect and understanding in relationships, fostering a sense of safety and security. As psychologist Dr. Henry Cloud noted, "Having clear boundaries is essential to a healthy, balanced lifestyle" and are fundamental for achieving personal growth and fulfilling connections.[35]

By recognizing the importance of boundaries, we can create a balanced life that honors our own needs while fostering healthier interactions with others. If you want to learn more about setting boundaries in your life, in your business, and your marriage, I strongly recommend the book *Boundaries: When to Say Yes, How to Say No to Take Control of Your Life* by Dr. Henry Cloud and Dr. John Townsend.

Setting boundaries is essential for healthy relationships and well-being. Here are a few examples of how that might look in the real world:

- When it comes to **time boundaries**, be clear about availability, such as saying, "I can only stay for an hour," or asking for notice in advance if someone will be late.

- **Energy boundaries** matter too—if you're unable to help, a response like "I don't have the energy right now, but this resource might be useful" keeps interactions respectful.

- **Emotional boundaries** help protect your mental health. If someone is venting and you're overwhelmed, a gentle but firm "I want to support you, but I don't have the emotional capacity to listen right now" can help.

- **Personal space boundaries** are important, too. If someone's behavior feels intrusive, expressing discomfort and setting consequences, like leaving, may be necessary.

- **Topical boundaries** can come into play in conversation. A direct "I'm not willing to discuss this right now" can shut down unwanted topics. Similarly, inappropriate remarks can be met with "I don't find that funny." If a discussion becomes too forceful, saying "I respect your opinion, but please don't push it on me" can reinforce your stance.

Even in digital spaces, boundaries apply. If someone posts something that makes you uncomfortable, a simple "I'd prefer if you didn't share that" sets a clear expectation. Though setting boundaries may feel uncomfortable, doing so fosters healthier, more respectful relationships in every aspect of life.

Setting boundaries is often misunderstood as being cruel or selfish, but in reality, it's a vital aspect of maintaining mental and emotional health. Boundaries allow you to define your personal space and protect your emotional well-being, ultimately fostering healthier relationships.

The opposite of a healthy relationship is a toxic one, and toxic relationships remind me of a documentary I once watched about the indigenous people of Borneo, some of the last remaining hunters who use poisoned darts. These hunters move stealthily beneath the jungle canopy, carrying blowguns loaded with small darts dipped in the deadly mucus of poison dart frogs. They silently stalk a monkey high above in the trees, shooting dart after dart at it. The sting of each dart is minor, not enough to drive the monkey to flee, but over time the poison accumulates, gradually disrupting the transmission of nerve signals to muscles. Eventually, this leads to cardiac failure, causing the monkey to fall into the waiting arms of the patient hunter.

In a similar way, a toxic relationship can feel like being struck by poisoned darts. The barbs and jabs from this person may not seem overwhelmingly painful at first, but over time, their toxicity builds up, accumulating in ways that can cause severe, lasting harm.

Toxic relationships come in many forms, each involving recurring, unhealthy patterns that can drain one or both partners emotionally, mentally, or physically. Toxic relationships come in various forms, but they generally involve behaviors or dynamics that negatively impact one or both people involved. Here are some common examples:

- **Controlling and Manipulative Behavior**: One person tries to control the other's actions, decisions, or even thoughts, often using guilt, threats, or pressure. This can make the other person feel powerless and unable to be themselves.

- **Excessive Criticism and Put-Downs**: In toxic relationships, criticism goes beyond constructive feedback. One person may constantly put the other down, undermining their self-esteem and making them feel unworthy or incapable.

- **Jealousy and Possessiveness**: While jealousy is normal to some extent, in toxic relationships it can become all-consuming. One partner may feel entitled to control or monitor the other, leading to constant accusations, snooping, or isolation.

- **Lack of Respect for Boundaries**: Boundaries are essential in healthy relationships, but in toxic ones, one partner may disregard or dismiss the other's needs, feelings, or limits, pushing them to do things they're uncomfortable with.

- **Emotional Neglect or Withdrawal**: Emotional neglect occurs when one partner consistently ignores the other's emotional needs, often refusing to provide support, affection, or attention. This can leave one person feeling lonely, unsupported, and unimportant.

- **Gaslighting**: This involves one person manipulating the other into doubting their own perceptions, memories, or reality. It's often used to gain control, make the other person feel inferior, or deflect responsibility.

- **Constant Drama and Turmoil**: In some relationships, there's a constant cycle of conflict, break-ups, and reconciliations. This instability can be exhausting, causing emotional distress and confusion.

- **Codependency**: In a codependent relationship, one person often feels responsible for the other's happiness and well-being, leading to an unhealthy reliance where individual needs and growth are sacrificed for the relationship.

- **Disregard for Personal Growth**: In a toxic relationship, one partner may discourage or belittle the other's ambitions or growth, whether it's about careers, hobbies, or personal development.

- **Physical or Emotional Abuse**: Any form of abuse, whether it's physical violence, emotional manipulation, or verbal attacks, is a serious sign of a toxic relationship. Abuse harms self-esteem, mental health, and sometimes even physical health.

Recognizing these toxic patterns can be the first step toward setting boundaries or making necessary changes for your well-being.

Ultimately, setting boundaries is not about shutting others out; it's about creating a healthy environment for ourselves and others. The mantra I use when wanting to set boundaries without being overly cruel or harsh is "Whitney, say what you mean; mean what you say; but don't say it mean."

MEN UNDER PRESSURE: RANDY'S STORY

When Randy, a man in his mid-thirties, first talked about his family struggles, his smile was as strained as forced small talk during a root canal procedure at the dental office. Beneath that façade was someone entangled in family expectations and unmet needs. Little did he know his story would soon become a masterclass in setting boundaries and reclaiming his autonomy.

Picture this: a boisterous Italian-American family, led by an extremely domineering matriarch who could control, manipulate, and guilt-trip not only her children but also her grandchildren. Randy's grandmother conducted this dysfunctional orchestra like a maestro, with Randy as the golden grandchild—showered with her approval while his cousins faded into the background for not bending to her every whim.

"I never wanted to disappoint her," Randy admitted quietly. "It controlled my whole life. I couldn't even say no when she piled groceries in my arms, more than I could carry on the train."

Growing up in a manipulative household didn't just erode Randy's self-confidence—it infiltrated his entire mindset, affecting every aspect of his life. He struggled to set personal limits, leaving him at the mercy of others' demands, and often found himself in toxic, one-sided relationships—attracting partners who treated him more like a servant than an equal. Randy also faced decision paralysis, where even simple choices like picking out an ice cream flavor could trigger anxiety. On top of all that, he was addicted to approval, chasing validation in a vicious and painful cycle.

Randy's transformation began when he made the brave decision to set boundaries, starting with his grandmother. It wasn't easy—initially, the thought of standing up to her terrified him—but slowly, he gained confidence and freedom. His journey started with small steps, like saying "no" to extra helpings at family dinners—a major feat in an Italian household. Though Nonna was shocked by his refusal, she eventually respected it when he stood his ground and refused to be bullied, as he had been so many times before.

Today, Randy is happier and more at ease with himself. He no longer feels the need to play the role of the "Golden Child."

Randy ultimately learned to empathize with his family without sacrificing his newfound independence. He studied how to establish boundaries, realizing they were essential for his well-being. His transformation from codependency to self-empowerment wasn't just a personal victory—it became a beacon of hope for anyone stuck in unhealthy family dynamics. With the right tools, courage, and a bit of humor, anyone can break free from the chains of codependency and rewrite their own story.

BOUNDARIES IN ACTION

Returning from Sierra Tucson with my newfound understanding of boundaries, I finally felt empowered to use my voice to advocate for myself. In life, we all have people we love spending time with, but we also have those who seem to drain the very essence out of us (for a vivid visual, refer to the 1982 movie *The Dark Crystal*).

When faced with invitations to events or activities that I, or my family, don't want to participate in, I learned to respond with honesty and respect. For example, I might say, "Your event sounds wonderful, but it doesn't work for me and my family, so we won't be able to attend." This response typically led to one of two outcomes.

The first, and easiest, was when the person replied with something like, "Oh, no worries! I hope we can have you join us next time."

The second outcome, however, was more challenging—when the person questioned or pushed back against my boundary. This could quickly escalate into hurt feelings, blame, or even burned bridges. For example, if someone said, "Whitney, I want to invite you to join my fight club," I might respond with, "Thank you for the kind invitation to your super-violent and destructive group, but that doesn't work for me or my family. Sorry."

If they replied with, "What?! Are you too good for us? Who do you think you are? If you were my friend, you'd come with me!"—or worse, added gaslighting or name-calling—I'd have two options:

- Option one: cave in and join the fight club to avoid confrontation.
- Option two: stand my ground.

I've learned to choose the latter. I might say, "Look, I'm going to be honest. I don't enjoy spending time with you. We're not that close, and I think this fight club is too extreme for me. Please don't send me any more invites like this. If you do, I'll need to sever our relationship."

If a family member is pressuring me into something I don't want to do, I could take a softer but still firm approach, such as "Listen, I love you, but I'm not on board with this plan. We're sitting this one out—maybe next time." Alternatively, I might say, "We're not interested in doing that. Please stop inviting us to your annual eggnog chugging contest. It's gross."

Staying firm in my boundaries protects me and keeps me safe mentally and emotionally. If someone can't respect your boundaries, maybe reconsider your relationship with them.

> **"Boundaries are the distance at which I can love you and me simultaneously."**
> —PRENTIS HEMPHILL

WHAT'S NEXT?

The truth is that even if you take all of these foundational steps—you take care of your body and mind, you get your financial house in order, you practice healthy communication and set healthy boundaries—sometimes you still need more help. There's no shame in that. In Part 3, we'll go there...as always, together.

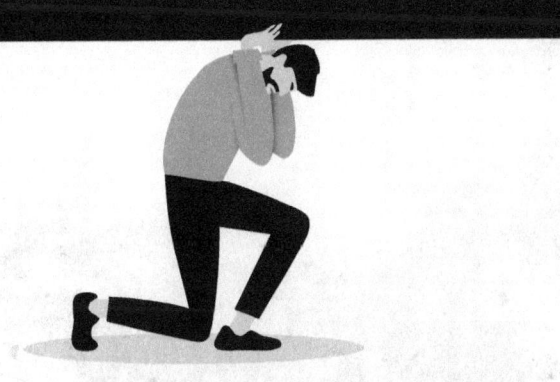

PART THREE
UP TO MY
NECK

ELEVEN

THE COURAGE TO SHARE

"You guys know about my ADHD diagnosis," I said to my siblings one Sunday evening over dinner. "But I've also been struggling with depression, and..."

My voice trailed off. How would they react? The conversation itself was long overdue, but I was still nervous.

But to my surprise, as soon as I started talking about my own experiences, my siblings began to open up as well. Turns out, some of them had been dealing with their own ADHD and depression issues for years and had even been prescribed medication to help manage their symptoms. We didn't realize at the time that there's a strong genetic component to many of these conditions, but now we know, and as G.I. Joe famously said, "Knowing is half the battle."

How had I not known about this before? How had we all been struggling in silence, too ashamed or afraid to talk about what we were going through?

As we continued to talk, I realized that my siblings had felt the same way I had—that there was a stigma around mental health issues, and that admitting to needing help was a sign of weakness.

Something amazing happened when we started to have these conversations. Suddenly, we all felt a little less alone. A little less broken. A little less ashamed. We realized that we'd been carrying these burdens by ourselves for far too long and that by sharing our stories with each other, we could start to heal and move forward.

And by opening up to my siblings and my loved ones, I realized that I didn't have to go through it alone anymore. I had a support system, a network of people who understood what I was going through and who were there to cheer me on every step of the way.

This newfound openness with my family laid the groundwork for overcoming another hurdle—dismantling the shame.

"Your story is the key that can unlock someone else's prison."

—UNKNOWN

SHARING MY STORY

No longer working as an orthodontist or as the chief clinical officer of Risas, I had a lot more time on my hands. I would spend lots of time with my kids, our animals, taking care of the house, and, of course, working on my beloved classic cars. I also spent countless hours pondering how I'd become a pathetic loser with no future. A has-been, washed-up, burned-out fool who felt so full of shame that I didn't know what to do next in my life. (Turns out I still needed to work on my self-talk.)

Looking for inspiration, I reached out to a close friend of mine I'd met in college, the now famous YouTuber Mark Rober. As of today my buddy Mark has more than 63 million subscribers to his unbelievably entertaining kid-friendly science channel, and my son and I had the unique pleasure of being in one of his videos (*How to Cheer the Loudest Using Science*...I'm the guy in the "Local Sports Team" T-shirt). A former NASA engineer turned YouTuber is not a normal career path, and I knew he'd have some good advice for me and my new path.

Mark has dealt with his own demons as he mourned the loss of his amazing mother to cancer at an early age, something he's shared on his channel in the past. Over the years since graduating from BYU together in 2004, we'd have brainstorming sessions on ways to go to the next level in our prospective careers, and I had a good feeling that he'd come through for me yet again. As we talked and I shared where I was in my personal and professional life, he listened very intently. He didn't interrupt me, staying quiet and letting me speak. I could tell his mental gears were turning, and he was engaged in thinking of ways of helping me in his own special way. At the end of my story, he was quiet for a long moment, then he said something that resonated deeply with my eighties-video-game-loving inner child.

While I was expecting him to commiserate with me and agree that my life was now terrible and hopeless, instead he knocked my socks off with his advice.

"Whitney, don't take this the wrong way, but this is such an exciting time in your life! It's like you've just started playing the Nintendo game *The Legend of Zelda* again for the very first time. You get a chance to choose your adventures and path all over again, to hit the reset button but as an adult, to experience the journey of building something completely new once again in your life. What a gift!"

It wasn't until he framed it that way that I began to see the possibilities of how I could use these experiences to truly help others. To think *I* could be the courageous hero Link once again, go on a new adventure, and collect incredible experiences as I rescued Princess Zelda from the grip of the evil Ganon! (Uh...I mean, helping other men tackle their mental health issues.) Mark was right. It truly was a gift. I'm incredibly grateful for Mark. He's not only a good friend but also a fierce advocate for autism awareness who has made huge leaps and strides in that arena to help us know how we can better understand those on the spectrum, like his own son.

My new journey took another interesting direction the day I had a heart-to-heart talk while hiking with my good friend Brandan, who encouraged me to share my story with the world via a podcast. He helped me recognize that I had a unique opportunity to speak with authority on the subject of men's mental health. A Brazilian Jiu-Jitsu World's gold medal winner and podcaster himself (*Make the Difference*), he assured me that it would be healing and helpful in ways I never imagined. He was right.

I first started sharing my mental health journey in August of 2020, with my podcast named *The Wright Talk*. I was worried people would think I was crazy. But then I realized, if they're thinking that, they're probably correct. Who in their right mind would willingly bare their soul to the world like this? But I found that the more openly I talked about my mental health issues, the more people would come to me for advice on steps they can take to heal from their own issues. In the end, I took the podcast down for personal reasons, but also because I was beginning to feel trapped by it. As you'll recall, I don't like feeling trapped whatsoever. But have no fear, I've included many of my guest's stories and basically the highlight reel of the podcast in this book, so you aren't missing anything juicy. Who knows, maybe I'll start a new podcast after this book is published. As Virginia Graham famously said, "I have the perfect face...for radio."

As I began to share more openly, I realized there was a deeper purpose behind it all. Sharing our stories is one of the most powerful things we can do when it comes to mental health. It's like shining a light into the darkest corners of our minds, exposing the shame and stigma that have been lurking there for far too long. And it isn't easy. It takes a level of vulnerability and courage that most people never have to muster in their entire lives.

But when we do share our stories, when we open up about our struggles and our triumphs, something incredible happens. We start to realize that we're not alone, that there are countless others out there who have faced similar challenges and came out the other side. And suddenly, the shame starts to lose its power. It's like we've pulled back the curtain on the great and powerful Oz, only to find a scared little man hiding behind a screen.

That's why dismantling the shame surrounding mental health is so crucial. For far too long, we've been told that mental illness is something to be ashamed of, something to hide away and never speak of. But the truth is, mental health challenges are just as real and valid as any physical ailment. And the more we talk about and normalize them, the less power that shame has over us. This realization led me to understand the importance of vulnerability in our journey to healing.

It's like the old saying goes—sunlight is the best disinfectant. And when it comes to mental health, shining a light on our struggles is the best way to start healing. It's not always easy, and it's not always comfortable, but it's always worth it. I know this firsthand because I've been on my own journey of sharing my experiences and encouraging open discussions about mental health. There have been moments of incredible vulnerability, moments where I've felt like I was standing naked in front of a crowd of strangers. But there have also been moments of profound connection, moments where I've seen the light of recognition and understanding in someone else's eyes.

And that's what keeps me going—the knowledge that by sharing my story, I might just be making a difference in someone else's life. That by being open and honest about my own struggles, I might just be giving someone else the courage to do the same.

This is why personal stories are so powerful—they create bridges where walls once stood.

> **"You can't go back and change the beginning, but you can start where you are and change the ending."**
> —C.S. LEWIS

CONNECTION THROUGH PERSONAL STORIES

Let's talk about the meat and potatoes of this whole sharing business—the personal stories themselves. Now, I know what some of you might be thinking: *Whitney, I'm not some fancy-pants writer or public speaker. I don't have any grand tales of heroism or triumph to share.* Every single one of us has a story worth sharing, no matter how big or small it may seem.

Dr. Brené Brown's research on vulnerability suggests that sharing personal stories can lead to greater connection and self-acceptance through several mechanisms:

- **Social Support**: Sharing creates a sense of connection and belonging, reducing feelings of isolation often associated with anxiety and low self-esteem. Strong social support networks have been shown to buffer against stress and improve overall mental well-being.

- **Emotional Processing**: Talking about experiences and feelings help you process emotions more effectively, gain perspective, and develop healthier coping mechanisms.

- **Validation**: Sharing personal struggles can lead to feeling understood and accepted, potentially boosting self-worth and confidence.

- **Normalization**: Hearing others share similar experiences can help you feel less alone and reduce feelings of shame or inadequacy.

- **Cognitive Reframing**: Discussing experiences with others can help you reframe your thoughts and perspectives, leading to a more positive self-image and reduced anxiety.

Sharing experiences and emotions can help reduce anxiety and improve self-esteem.[36] And it's in this sharing that we find the true power of vulnerability. Brené Brown's books are fantastic and have played a large role in my ability to speak openly about these issues. I strongly recommend checking out her collection.

HOW TO DO YOUR PART TO HELP REDUCE STIGMA

The power of sharing our stories goes beyond just helping individuals—it can also have a profound impact on society as a whole.

Remember the stigma surrounding men's mental health that we talked about at the beginning of the book? Every time we share our experiences with mental health challenges, we're chipping away at that stigma. We're showing the world that mental illness is not a personal failing but a medical condition that deserves the same compassion and understanding as any other.

And the more we chip away at that stigma and the more we normalize conversations about mental health, the easier it becomes for others to seek help when they need it. We're not just helping ourselves by sharing our stories—we're helping to create a world where mental health is taken seriously and where those who struggle are met with empathy and support instead of judgment and shame.

These changes start with simple, everyday conversations—those in-person moments that can change a life. Here are some examples of stories you can share.

IN-PERSON CONVERSATIONS

I know the idea of sharing your personal story can be daunting, but it doesn't have to be a grand public display. Some of the most powerful conversations I've had about mental health have been the ones that happened in private, with only one other person. There's something about the intimacy of those in-person conversations that allows for a level of vulnerability and connection that's hard to find anywhere else.

I remember one conversation in particular with a close friend who, unbeknownst to me, had been struggling with depression for years. We were having lunch together, just chatting about life, when he suddenly got quiet and bravely said, "I haven't been doing so well lately."

At that moment, I knew I had a choice. I could either brush it off and change the subject, or I could lean in and listen. Knowing the pain that comes from suffering in silence, I leaned in. I asked him to tell me more, to share what he was going through. And as he spoke, I could see the relief wash over his face. He started to become emotional, and his tears showed me just how bad it was for him. It was like he'd been carrying this heavy burden for so long, and the act of finally sharing it with someone else made it feel a little lighter.

Sometimes, though, sharing means stepping onto a bigger stage.

PUBLIC SPEAKING ENGAGEMENTS

I've had the privilege of speaking at conferences and events about my own journey with mental health, and it's a rush like no other. There's something about standing up in front of a crowd of strangers and baring your soul that's both terrifying and exhilarating.

I remember the first time I gave a speech about my struggles with anxiety and depression. I was shaking like a leaf, my palms sweaty and my heart racing. But as I started to speak, as I saw the nods of recognition and the tears in people's eyes, I realized that I was tapping into something powerful. I was giving a voice to the struggles that so many of us face but so few of us talk about.

And after the speech, when person after person came up to me and shared their own stories, I knew that I had made a difference. I had shown them that they weren't alone, that there was no shame in their struggles, and that there was always hope for a better tomorrow.

But it's not just about telling our own stories; it's also about encouraging others to share theirs.

ENCOURAGING OTHERS TO SHARE THEIR PATHS

I know what you might be thinking: *Whitney, I'm not some big-shot influencer or celebrity. How can I possibly encourage others to share their stories?* Well let me tell you a secret—you don't need a million followers or a fancy title to make a difference. All you need is a willingness to lead by example and create safe spaces for others to share their truths.

Creating safe spaces is just the beginning, because while it's important for people to feel comfortable sharing their stories, it's equally crucial to take proactive steps to support them. Simply saying "It's okay to not be okay" isn't enough. We need to go further by offering concrete resources and support, such as connecting individuals with mental health professionals, providing information on coping strategies, and fostering a community that actively encourages and celebrates their progress. This holistic approach not only helps people feel heard and understood but also empowers them to seek the help they need and sustain their mental health journey.

And one of the most powerful ways to encourage others is by leading through our own example. If you would like to share your mental health success story with me and many other Men Under Pressure, please go to **menunderpressure** **.com**. Who knows? Your story may be the key that unlocks the healing in other men looking for guidance and hope.

LEADING BY EXAMPLE

When it comes to dismantling the shame surrounding mental health, actions speak louder than words. Every time you share your own story, every time you open up about your struggles and your triumphs, you're sending a powerful message to those around you. You're showing them that it's okay to be vulnerable, that there's no shame in struggling, and that seeking help is a sign of strength, not weakness.

And here's the thing—people are watching. Even if you don't realize it, there are people in your life who look up to you, who see you as a role model and a source of inspiration. And when they see you being open and honest about your mental health journey, it gives them permission to do the same.

TWELVE

PRIORITIZING HEALING AND HAPPINESS

"You know, Mr. Whitney, I have never told anyone about this since moving to the US, but when I was a child, my dad verbally abused me."

These words came from my barber, Abraham, whom I've been going to for many years. We often talk about all kinds of topics—sometimes even in Spanish, as he's from Nicaragua. This topic, though, had never come up before. I was in shock, meeting his watery eyes in the mirror in front of us.

I felt a wave of sadness. Suddenly, a look of determination seemed to wash over him, and he continued, "No, it was more than verbal abuse...he physically abused me as well." He rolled up his sleeve to show me scars on his arm, wounds inflicted by his father when he was a young teen. He told me his legs and back were also covered in similar scars.

As the oldest child, Abraham had borne the brunt of his father's rage. Most of his scars, he explained, came from his father whipping him with barbed wire. I was in shock. With a far-off look in his eyes, he recounted a story he had never shared with anyone, telling me he eventually ran away at fifteen to live with his uncle in the US.

He was vulnerable because I was vulnerable first, illustrating this true connective power. Moments before, I'd blurted out that I was writing a book.

He'd looked at me, surprised, as if to see if I was kidding. I reassured him that I was indeed writing a mental health guide for men. With genuine curiosity, he asked, "How did you decide to do that? Have you ever written a book before?" I replied, "No, I haven't, but when I was a kid, I was sexually abused, and it really messed me up. I eventually developed depression and anxiety and was having panic attacks, which is why I had to stop practicing orthodontics. I hope that by sharing my story, other men will feel safe to do the same and start healing from their wounds."

That's when he paused his clippers and told me his own story, right there in the barbershop.

This story illustrates that we never know what people are going through, and we never know what connections we can form when we show up with vulnerability and compassion. Especially as men, we need more spaces like that for us in the world. When we open up about our struggles, our fears, and our darkest moments, we aren't just putting ourselves out there— we're inviting others to do the same. We're creating a space where it's okay to not be okay, where it's okay to admit that we're struggling and need help.

And that vulnerability? It's like a magic key that unlocks the hearts and minds of those around us. Beyond personal healing, our vulnerability plays a crucial role in breaking down societal barriers. When we're vulnerable, we give others permission to be vulnerable, too. We show them that they're not alone, that there's no shame in struggling, and that there's always hope for a brighter tomorrow.

> "To share your weakness is to make yourself vulnerable; to make yourself vulnerable is to show your strength."
> —CRISS JAMI

WHEN IT'S TIME TO GET HELP

When it comes to seeking professional help (and in my case, taking medication), we have to feel safe and supported in the process. Whether it's with a therapist, a psychiatrist, or any other mental health professional, we need to know that we can be vulnerable and honest without fear of judgment or rejection. We need to feel like our needs and boundaries are being respected and that our healing is the top priority.

That's why it's so important for us to create those safe spaces, both for ourselves and for others. Whether it's in therapy, in support groups, or just in our everyday conversations with loved ones, we need to be intentional about fostering an environment of openness, empathy, and acceptance. We do this by allowing others to share their stories without interrupting them or trying to one-up their traumas with your own. Even worse is asking them to stop talking because we don't want to hear it or telling them to just "man up." You can't just "rub some dirt on it" and "tough" your way out of these issues.

They need to be coaxed out in a safe environment so shame doesn't come sweeping in to bury those traumatic shards even deeper. Everyone struggles in one way or another. *Everyone.* By remembering this, we can listen and support others without becoming a stumbling block on their way to healing. When we feel safe to speak our truths and share our struggles, that's when real healing can begin.

I emphasize the importance of fostering an environment of openness, empathy, and nonjudgment through several actionable steps:

- **Active Listening and Validation**: When someone comes to me with their struggles, I make it a point to listen intently and validate their feelings without interrupting or offering unsolicited advice. This approach helps make the person feel heard and understood.

- **Encouraging Professional Help**: Instead of trying to solve the person's problems myself, I guide them toward professional help. This involves offering to help them find a professional and supporting them in taking that step.

- **Setting Boundaries**: I stress the importance of setting boundaries to avoid becoming overwhelmed by someone else's struggles. This includes being honest about the extent to which I can help and ensuring that I don't become a crutch for the person, which can hinder their healing process.

- **Creating Safe Spaces**: I highlight the need for creating environments where people feel safe to share their experiences without fear of judgment. This involves being empathetic and understanding that mental health issues are real and not something people choose to have.

- **Promoting Open Conversations**: I encourage open and honest conversations about mental health to destigmatize it. Sharing personal stories and experiences can help others feel less isolated and more willing to seek help.

By implementing these practices, we can create a supportive and nonjudgmental environment that fosters openness and empathy, making it easier for individuals to seek and receive the help they need.

But we can't do it alone—and that's where the power of a supportive community comes in. When we surround ourselves with people who understand what we're going through, who can offer encouragement and inspiration, and who can remind us that we're not alone in our struggles, it makes all the difference in the world.

Whether it's a formal support group or just a few close friends who have been through similar challenges, having a network of people who get it can be a lifeline. They can help us to see the progress we've made, even when we feel like we're stuck in quicksand. They can offer practical advice and resources or just a listening ear when we need to vent. And most importantly, they can remind us that we're not broken or defective, that we're worthy of love and support and healing, no matter what.

Whether you're just starting out on your mental health journey or you've been at it for years, know that you are seen, you are valued, and you are never, ever alone. So keep going, keep fighting, keep leaning on each other and creating those safe spaces for growth and vulnerability. And who knows—maybe one day, you'll look back on this chapter of your life and see it as the turning point, the moment when you decided to stop suffering in silence and start speaking your truth. When we choose to prioritize our own healing and happiness, the rest will fall into place.

> "Your willingness to share your story can open the door for someone else to heal."
> —IYANLA VANZANT

MENTAL HEALTH RESOURCES AND SUPPORT OPTIONS

If you're struggling with mental health issues, know that help is available. Here's a list of resources in the United States that can provide support:

- National Suicide Prevention Lifeline
    - Call 1-800-273-8255 (Available 24/7)
    - Website: suicidepreventionlifeline.org

- Crisis Text Line
    - Text HOME to 741741 (Available 24/7)
    - Website: crisistextline.org

- National Alliance on Mental Illness (NAMI)
    - Helpline: 1-800-950-NAMI (6264)
    - Website: nami.org
    - Offers support groups, education programs, and advocacy

- Substance Abuse and Mental Health Services Administration (SAMHSA)
    - National Helpline: 1-800-662-HELP (4357)
    - Website: samhsa.gov
    - Provides referrals to local treatment facilities, support groups, and community-based organizations

ONLINE THERAPY PLATFORMS

- BetterHelp: betterhelp.com
- Talkspace: talkspace.com

MENTAL HEALTH APPS

- Calm: Meditation and sleep app
- Headspace: Mindfulness and meditation app
- Moodfit: Mood tracking and mental health tools
- Insight Timer: Hundreds of free guided meditations

ONLINE COMMUNITIES

- Reddit's r/mentalhealth: reddit.com/r/mentalhealth
- 7 Cups: 7cups.com—free emotional support and online therapy

LOCAL RESOURCES

- Community mental health centers: Search for centers in your area
- University counseling centers: For students, check your school's website
- Employee assistance programs (EAPs): Check with your employer about available mental health services

"Beautiful are those whose brokenness
gives birth to transformation and wisdom."
—JOHN GREEN

BE A CHAMPION FOR YOURSELF AND OTHERS

We've covered the transformative power of sharing personal stories, the importance of vulnerability, and the impact of creating safe spaces. Sharing our experiences can reduce stigma, foster community, and encourage others to seek help.

I challenge you to take the leap and share your own mental health journey with someone you trust. Your story has the power to inspire and provide hope to others. Remember, you don't need to be a big-shot influencer to make a difference; your voice matters.

Lead by example, create safe spaces for open dialogue, and support those around you. Celebrate every victory, no matter how small. Together, we can create a world where mental health is taken seriously and everyone is met with compassion and support.

Let this be your rallying cry, your call to action, your reminder that your story matters and your voice has power. Let this be the moment where you decide to step out of the shadows and into the light—not just for yourself but for everyone around you.

Together, we can dismantle shame, encourage open discussion, and create a more compassionate world—one story at a time. So let's get out there and start sharing our truths like the nitty-gritty mental health warriors we are! Need a baby step idea? Consider writing down the names of three people you trust and whom you could open up to. Look at that list every day—as many days as it takes—until you have the courage to have that conversation with one of them. Then, keep going.

And remember—if all else fails, just picture me cheering you on from the sidelines, like a sidewalk sign spinner twirling a massive sign saying, "You Got This!" Because if there's one thing I know for sure, it's that men are capable of amazing things—and I'll be here rooting for you every step of the way.

So step into the light and share your truth.

Let's dismantle shame, one story at a time.

JOIN SUPPORT GROUPS

A s I settled into life at Sierra Tucson, it quickly became clear that everyone was fighting their own unseen battles. John's story stood out—a tale of addiction, despair, and, ultimately, redemption that illustrated how far one can fall and still find a way back. I first locked eyes with John across the sun-drenched courtyard, both of us newly admitted and looking more like discarded marionettes than the successful professionals we once were. The transformation I witnessed in him over the coming weeks was nothing short of miraculous.

MEN UNDER PRESSURE: JOHN'S STORY

John's journey serves as a testament to the raw power of facing one's demons head-on. Picture Philadelphia in the late seventies: John's father, a stern disciplinarian, cast a shadow over his childhood while his mother tried to compensate with warmth.

"My father made me feel lesser," John admitted during one of our late-night chats. "He made me feel stupid. But I had undiagnosed ADHD." This misdiagnosis shaped his self-image profoundly, leading him to struggle academically while his father dismissed his challenges as laziness.

At the tender age of twelve, John and a friend raided the liquor cabinet. That first sip was a revelation, marking the moment he found the magic elixir to quiet his inner turmoil. By high school, he was drinking heavily and playing the class clown to mask his insecurities. Fast forward a couple decades: John appeared to have it all—a thriving career, a loving wife, and three daughters. Yet beneath that polished exterior, his drinking had escalated into full-blown addiction, exacerbated by pills. "I knew what I was doing was killing me," he admitted, aware that his actions were hurting his family.

It was a classic case of an addict circling the drain. His wife, at her wit's end, began siphoning money from their accounts as a secret escape fund and went to Al-Anon for support. But John spiraled further, eventually moving out to an apartment where he spent a year curled up in the fetal position, with bottles of alcohol and Percocet by his side. He'd reached rock bottom.

Enter Sierra Tucson. Unlike his first rehab experience, which felt superficial, John was now determined to reclaim his life. He threw himself into recovery with the fervor of someone fighting for their very soul. EMDR therapy helped him process past traumas, while Alcoholics Anonymous (AA) kept him sober. The results were transformative: John has now been sober for over five years, rebuilding relationships and finding a new purpose in helping others battling addiction.

"I have three daughters," he shared, emotion thick in his voice. "I have letters from them—one from each of my sweet daughters—telling me I'm their hero."

John's journey is a powerful reminder that recovery is a lifelong commitment, requiring constant vigilance and self-awareness. As he put it, "Alcohol is cunning, baffling, powerful, and patient...I know it's waiting for me." To stay sober, John attends multiple AA support groups a week. He's now a sponsor for many recovering alcoholics and even helps run an AA group in the local prison. He's learned that by participating in support groups, he can stay sober, living just one day at a time.

His journey reminds us that it's never too late to rewrite your story. Healing may be grotesquely uncomfortable and downright terrifying at times, but on the other side of that fear is where real living begins—and in his case, it began in a support group right there in Sierra Tucson, in a chair next to mine.

> "Sometimes, reaching out and taking
> someone's hand is the beginning
> of a journey. At other times, it is
> allowing another to take yours."
> —VERA NAZARIAN

THE BEGINNER'S GUIDE TO THERAPY

This section feels a bit tricky to write, and here's why: If your car was running poorly and I suggested, "Just take it to a mechanic," you'd likely have follow-up questions, such as, "What type of mechanic do you recommend? Where can I find a good one? How much will the repair cost, and how long will it take?" While I can't answer all these questions, I can help you navigate the process of finding a therapist rather than just handing you a solution.

HOW TO FIND THE RIGHT THERAPIST

In my experience, there are several effective ways to find a good therapist. Often, when I share my struggles, the person I'm speaking with has either been to therapy themselves or knows someone who has and can recommend a therapist. Another route is to ask your medical professional for recommendations; when discussing your issues with your doctor or psychiatrist, ask if they can suggest a therapist. Additionally, searching

online can be invaluable—look up terms such as "male therapist" or "therapy for men" in your area and read reviews. Positive
reviews can be a strong indicator of a good fit. If you find a therapist with favorable feedback, visit their website to read their
bio and treatment philosophy. If it resonates with you, reach
out and schedule an appointment.

Typically, the first session with a therapist is longer than
subsequent visits. It's crucial to be as honest and vulnerable
as possible during this initial meeting, as it allows the therapist to understand your situation better. Pay attention to how
you feel with them: Do you feel comfortable, heard, and safe?
It's important to find someone who will listen and support your
progress. For my own traumatic past, I sought a therapist specializing in EMDR, but you might prefer someone who focuses
on CBT or even ketamine therapy.

EMDR is a structured therapy method that helps individuals
process traumatic experiences through eight phases, including
history taking, preparation, assessment, desensitization (using
bilateral stimulation), installation of positive beliefs, body scan,
closure, and re-evaluation. It's been shown to effectively treat
PTSD and other trauma-related conditions by helping individuals reprocess memories and lessen their emotional impact.

CBT is another structured, goal-oriented approach that
focuses on identifying and changing negative thought patterns and behaviors. It emphasizes the interconnectedness of
thoughts, feelings, and behaviors, aiming to improve emotional
well-being and coping strategies. CBT is commonly used for
various mental health issues, including anxiety, depression,

and stress, employing techniques like cognitive restructuring and behavioral activation. It's typically a short-term method and emphasizes practical skills for everyday life.

Ketamine therapy uses low doses of ketamine, a dissociative anesthetic, to treat conditions like depression, anxiety, and PTSD. Administered intravenously or via nasal spray, ketamine works quickly, often providing relief within hours, in contrast to traditional antidepressants that may take weeks. It's believed to enhance synaptic connections and promote neuroplasticity, benefiting those who haven't responded to other treatments. However, it should be conducted under medical supervision due to potential side effects and ongoing research into its long-term efficacy.

There are various treatment modalities available, and my aim isn't to overwhelm you. I simply want to highlight that many types of therapy all focus on similar goals: uncovering buried emotional pain and facilitating healing.

So step one in finding a good therapist is simply that—finding one. Take your time, trust your instincts, do your research, and then take the plunge. It may not be easy, but it will undoubtedly be worth it.

WHAT TO EXPECT IN A SESSION

Okay, so you've found a therapist—now what? The goal of therapy is to help you see aspects of your life that you might be overlooking, recognize patterns, identify past traumas, and equip you with tools to avoid manipulation or abuse. Your therapist becomes a mentor, healer, coach, and listening ear all rolled into one. They may ask difficult questions, such as "Tell me about your relationship with your father." In response, you might feel your heart race, your face flush, and your palms sweat. Your instinct might be to say, "It was okay," but your body tells a different story. A good therapist will pick up on these non-verbal cues and ask about your feelings: "Do you feel nervous talking about your dad? Is there a specific memory that comes to mind?" This is precisely what you hired them to do—explore your psyche to uncover the hidden pain of buried shards.

When they sense they've found something significant, they'll gently probe further to understand its depth and impact. Don't shut down or shy away from this process. Trust the journey; it may be painful, and you might cry or feel terrified, but these reactions are part of healing. Your body and mind need to release these buried shards, so lean into the discomfort. You're strong enough to face difficult situations. Do this for yourself— love yourself enough to heal. The alternative is to let these buried shards continue to poison you. Whatever it takes, get them out.

Once the shards are removed, it's time to heal. What does healing look like? It could involve establishing boundaries—like ensuring your mother-in-law doesn't take control of your home when she visits—or telling your boss that you won't respond to work emails after 5:00 p.m. It might also mean forgiving some-one who has hurt you and moving on from the pain. I've had to do this multiple times. My first major betrayal came from my abuser, whom I ultimately forgave. The toxic shards of hatred and resentment I constantly carried around with me were extremely burdensome, so I worked to remove them and let go of the past. This doesn't mean I have a relationship with him; I forgave the abusive behavior and moved on.

In business, I faced betrayal from a close friend whom I'd brought into our company. After years of working together, he betrayed my trust by opening up a direct competitor dental and orthodontic company that *very* closely resembled ours. He justified his actions to me, saying, "It's just business, Whitney, nothing personal." But it felt very personal to me. That betrayal sadly led to legal action and the end of our friendship.

Several years after that lawsuit, he reached out, asking to meet for breakfast. I was reluctant, but he assured me he wanted to apologize, which he did. I forgave him—but I didn't rekindle the relationship. The pain from that ordeal was too great to reopen. About a year after that breakfast, he contacted me again, hoping we could meet. His text read, "Hey, it looks like you stopped doing your podcast. I was a follower of it and really enjoyed your discussions on mental health. I'm starting to feel like I'm cracking under the pressure and wanted to talk if you're open to it."

I can't begin to describe how upset I was to receive that text. It felt like a betrayal, especially considering the similarity between his business model and ours and the fact that we're now direct competitors. I held off responding until I could talk to my wife. I expressed my anger and frustration with his request, and after listening to my rant, she calmly said, "Whitney, didn't you say you wouldn't wish what happened to you on *anyone*?"

I was both shocked and humbled by her response. She was right—I had said those exact words many times. So I agreed to meet with him.

During our meeting, it was clear he wasn't well. His health was deteriorating, and his eyes looked hollow—almost lifeless. He shared the toll that running a dental and orthodontic company had taken on him, describing the negative effects he was experiencing.

I told him I understood exactly how he felt. I offered advice, suggested steps he could take to regain his well-being, and wished him the best.

Six months later, I ran into him again, and he reported that he was prioritizing self-care and working with a life and business coach to stay on track. He humbly thanked me for my willingness to talk him through it and keep him from drowning in the abyss. The renewed hope I now saw in his eyes reassured me that I'd done the right thing...I'd helped another man under pressure.

Therapy helps you uncover what may be hiding in plain sight. Have you ever searched the fridge for something and couldn't find it, only to have someone point out that it's right in front of you? That's what a good therapist can do—they help you see what's obvious but overlooked. Maybe you're in an abusive relationship and don't understand why you feel so trapped. Perhaps you struggle with toxic shame or an addiction that you dismiss as a hobby. Whatever it is, trained therapists can help you recognize these issues and guide you toward a happier, healthier life.

I know therapy may be a financial burden, and your health insurance may not cover it. However, prioritizing your mental health will always pay off in the long run. Consider budgeting for these treatments or even taking on a part-time job to make it work. Ultimately, your most important responsibility is to take care of yourself so you can continue to provide for and protect your loved ones.

> **"Nothing ever goes away until it has taught us what we need to know."**
> —PEMA CHÖDRÖN

CONSIDERING MEDICATION

Through therapy, I learned to embrace my imperfections, which led me to reconsider taking medication. I used to believe that taking medication was a cop-out, a way to avoid the real work of therapy and self-improvement. However, I discovered that no amount of therapy or self-help reading could prevent my mental health from deteriorating, and that's exactly what happened to me.

It started slowly—just a bit more anxiety here and a touch more depression there. Before I knew it, I was engulfed in a full-blown mental health crisis, experiencing daily panic attacks accompanied by intense fear and physical symptoms like rapid heartbeat, shortness of breath, and dizziness. I felt like I was "losing my grip on reality," overwhelmed and unable to manage my emotions or situation. Getting out of bed became a struggle, and I felt like I was drowning in a sea of negative thoughts.

I tried to push through, relying on my usual methods of "toughing it out." But this time, no amount of positive self-talk or deep breathing could pull me out of the hole I was in. I realized I needed real help—not just the kind that comes from talking about my feelings for an hour each week. So, at my therapist's urging, I made an appointment with a psychiatrist who could evaluate my symptoms and guide my treatment.

Walking into that first appointment, I was incredibly nervous. I had always resisted the idea of medication, even when I'd taken ADHD meds in dental school, and I worried about what it meant to admit that I needed help again. However, my psychiatrist was kind and understanding, helping me see that there was no shame in seeking help, regardless of its form. Together, we decided that medication was the right choice for me. She prescribed an antidepressant and anti-anxiety medication, discussing potential side effects and what I could expect regarding symptom relief.

Even with my psychiatrist's reassurance, I struggled with the stigma surrounding medication. I felt as though I was admitting defeat, that I was somehow weak for needing a pill to function. Over time, I worked hard to overcome those negative beliefs, realizing that medication is just one tool in the mental health toolbox. I used a combination of therapeutic techniques, self-reflection, and challenging my ego to shift my perspective.

Here are some specific methods I employed:

- **Reading Eckhart Tolle's** *The Power of Now*: I started this book shortly after being admitted to Sierra Tucson, which introduced me to the concept of the ego as an alternate persona feeding false narratives. This realization helped me ignore the negative self-talk driven by my ego.

- **Challenging My Ego**: I actively confronted my ego, which often dismissed certain therapies as pointless. By setting my ego aside and being open to trying new practices—like group drum therapy, tai chi, and Tibetan singing bowl therapy—I discovered their unexpected benefits, allowing me to grow and heal.

- **Seeking Professional Guidance**: Emphasizing the importance of professional help, I understood that being diagnosed with specific disorders validated my experiences and provided a clear treatment path. This insight was crucial in overcoming the intense negative self-talk and shame I felt.

- **Practicing Mindfulness and Meditation**: Practicing mindfulness and meditation helped me stay present and manage my anxiety, offering essential tools for self-regulation.

I learned that medication isn't a magic bullet and doesn't replace therapy or lifestyle changes. For some people, including me, it can be a necessary part of the healing process. I had to let go of shame and judgment, accepting that my mental health is as important as my physical health and that seeking help for either is not a sign of weakness. Gradually, I began to see the benefits of medication in my life.

THE TRIFECTA: MEDICATION, THERAPY, AND LIFESTYLE CHANGES

It's important to understand that medication alone is rarely sufficient to address mental health issues. It's just one piece of the puzzle and works best in combination with therapy and lifestyle changes. That's why, even as I started medication, I continued working with my therapist and making daily changes to support my mental health. I continued exercising regularly and focused on eating a healthier diet and prioritizing self-care activities like meditation and journaling.

As I began to feel better, I started to see how all these elements fit together. Medication helped stabilize my mood and reduce anxiety, while therapy equipped me with the tools to address my underlying issues and develop healthier coping mechanisms. The lifestyle changes I made provided a foundation for overall wellness, supporting my ongoing healing. This holistic approach reminded me that prioritizing my well-being is essential every step of the way.

It wasn't always easy, and there were moments when I felt like I was taking two steps forward and one step back. For instance, uncovering hidden issues from my past with my therapist often meant facing yet another challenge to work through. But I kept going, kept putting one foot in front of the other, and maintained my belief that healing was possible—even on the darkest days.

Setbacks often arise from stressful events such as losing your job or going through a bad breakup, triggering negative thoughts and emotions. This might lead to increased anxiety and depression, resulting in feelings of shame, guilt, and disappointment, making me question my progress. During these times, I relied on my strong support system, my practice of self-compassion, my belief in my own healing, and my commitment to sticking with therapy and support groups. It wasn't easy, but boy, was it worth it.

Slowly but surely, I began to feel like myself again—not the old me, who was always trying to outrun pain and fear, but a new me—stronger, wiser, and more compassionate to myself and others.

My decision to start medication marked a turning point in my journey. I acknowledged that I needed help and that there was no shame in admitting it. This was a step toward prioritizing my well-being and happiness above all else.

If you're on the fence about therapy or medication, the most important thing is to remember that you're not alone. There's a community of people who have walked this path before you, who understand the pain and struggle, and who are cheering you on every step of the way. Keep going, keep fighting, and keep believing in yourself. With the right support and tools, anything is possible.

"You don't break an ankle and keep walking on it; you use a crutch so it can heal. Medicine can be a crutch until you're strong enough to heal on your own."

—SAVANNA SMITH

WHAT'S NEXT?

If you're struggling with your mental health and feel like you've tried everything with no success, know this: There's no shame in seeking help, whatever form it takes. Medication, therapy, and lifestyle changes are all valid and valuable tools in the pursuit of healing and wholeness.

So is inpatient therapy, though that's a step further. If you're already drowning, though, you need more direct, lifesaving interventions. In Part 4, I'm going to tell you about mine.

PART FOUR
DIVING DEEP

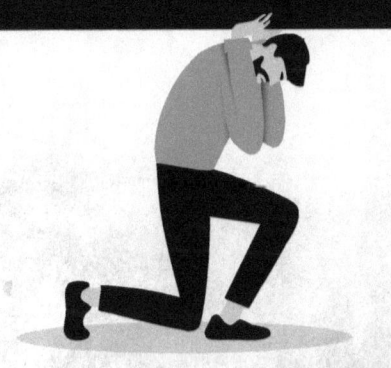

FOURTEEN

A NEW BEGINNING

"Hi there," I said to the receptionist at Sierra Tucson, attempting to lighten the mood. "I'm here to check myself in. My name's Whitney—like Whitney Houston, but I'm a guy."

She looked puzzled, clearly not expecting humor from someone admitting themselves to a mental health facility. I shrugged, adding, "I'm just trying to make you laugh to keep myself from crying. I'm freaking out here."

With that awkward icebreaker out of the way, I provided my information, my heart rate increasing as the reality set in. I'd reached my breaking point. The panic attacks, depression, and anxiety had taken over my life, and I could no longer pretend everything was okay. Remember? My psychiatrist had given me an ultimatum: Check into a thirty-day treatment facility, or she could no longer continue seeing me. It was time to face my demons head-on.

"Alrighty then!"

—ACE VENTURA, PET DETECTIVE

A SENSE OF SHAME

As I walked into the beautiful lobby of Sierra Tucson, a wave of shame washed over me. Here I was, a successful orthodontist and entrepreneur, reduced to seeking extreme help for my mental health. But there was no turning back now.

The intake process was thorough and somewhat humiliating. To ensure I wasn't bringing anything harmful into the facility, I was strip-searched, and any scars on my body were marked for monitoring. I felt completely exposed as I surrendered my belongings—my phone, wallet, keys, and clothes—before they placed me in a holding area. I wondered if this was what it felt like to go to jail; I now felt trapped in one. It was like shedding my old identity and stepping into a new, vulnerable chapter of my life.

That holding area, called "Desert Rose," was where I spent the first forty-eight hours being evaluated by psychiatrists, psychologists, and therapists alongside all the other patients being admitted. The staff aimed to determine the best course of treatment for me, but at the time, I felt out of place. I thought it was overkill—that my problems weren't as severe as those of other patients. I felt like a fish out of water, not some strung-out drug addict or alcoholic drying out for the first time.

As the days passed and I shed my ego, I realized this was exactly where I needed to be. I was just as broken as everyone else, even if I'd been in denial about it. So I surrendered to the process, determined to get the most out of the experience.

Little did I know this was just the beginning of a journey that would change my life forever. The forty-eight hour detox and intake process was merely a precursor to the real work ahead— an intensive exploration of my psyche through various therapy modalities. I was about to embark on a deep dive into my past traumas and present struggles, and it would take every ounce of courage I had to emerge on the other side. For the first time in a long time, I had hope that healing was possible.

The recovery process was grueling, both physically and mentally. Between individual and group sessions, I was in therapy for almost ten hours a day. Those thirty days of intensely focused work laid the foundation for my recovery. Despite my initial discomfort, I knew that to maximize my time at Sierra Tucson, I needed not just to surrender but to fully commit to the program—"trust the process," as they say. Embracing it was not just about physical cleansing; it was about clearing the mental and emotional clutter that had accumulated over the years.

EMBRACING THE DETOX PROGRAM

From that moment, I embraced the treatment program as if it were school. Each week came with a planned schedule, so I always knew what I'd be doing and where I needed to be. Breakfast was at 6:30, and from there, the day unfolded. There were a few planned breaks, but for the most part, they ensured I utilized my time wisely.

Every morning, all the men in our lodge (or housing unit) gathered to discuss our goals for the day, and in the evening, we recapped our progress and what we'd learned. Afterward, we had personal time to play ping-pong, journal, or read before lights out. Those meetings were critical in helping me realize that everyone struggles and just wants to feel healthy and loved.

It was refreshing to unplug from the real world for a while and focus on healing.

One thing was certain, though: A one-size-fits-all approach wasn't going to cut it. Sierra Tucson employed a diverse array of individual, group, and experiential therapies tailored to each patient's needs. For me, that meant a combination of one-on-one sessions, group processing, somatic work to reconnect my mind and body, inner-child therapy to heal my wounded younger self, and even equine therapy in the desert landscape. Whether it was coloring, painting, or meditation, if it could facilitate healing, they offered it. I attended every group, course, and therapy session available; after all, I'm an overachieving workaholic.

But the real turning point for me was EMDR. By the end of my time at Sierra Tucson, I felt fundamentally transformed. I felt like I'd been thoroughly pulled apart, cleaned, and put back together—still me, but a new and improved version, with long-buried pieces finally reintegrated.

STRONGER TOGETHER

Beyond the therapies, being immersed in the Sierra Tucson environment was hugely impactful. Depending on individual needs, patients were housed in different accommodations spread across the beautiful desert campus. I quickly bonded with my housemates, all of whom were there due to some form of trauma, whether overt and violent or insidious and unseen.

At first glance, my fellow residents seemed very different. There was the high-powered attorney who looked like he could chew nails for breakfast, the former CEO with a mask-like expression hiding her inner turmoil, and the artist whose bright, colorful outfits belied her fragility. But as we opened up, it became clear we all wore similar façades to obscure our brokenness.

Some of us were wrestling with deep-seated psychiatric conditions or hormonal imbalances that had gone unchecked for years. Others were tormented by addictions—chasing the next dopamine hit from alcohol, drugs, gambling, sex, or other vices. But strip away the symptoms, and we were all driven by unprocessed, *unhealed trauma.*

I'll never forget Michael, a hulking figure whose menacing appearance suggested he'd just been released from prison. My first thought was to hope I didn't anger him. Yet, as his tough exterior softened, a painfully shy and sensitive soul emerged. One group session, he broke down in wrenching sobs as he opened up about the sexual abuse he'd endured as a child. Here was a man whom I'd assumed was a perpetrator; in reality, he was a survivor mustering every ounce of courage just to exist.

As I witnessed Michael and others confront their innermost agonies, I felt awe and kinship. We were a motley crew, thrown together by fate and circumstance, yet we were somehow stronger together than any of us could have been alone. Our unique paths converged at Sierra Tucson for an intensive immersion in psychic archaeology—excavating the deep pains, traumas, and destructive patterns that had held us hostage.

But excavation was only the first phase of reckoning. Having unearthed our wounds, Sierra's next pivotal role was to provide the tools and nurturing environment necessary for actual healing. While the road ahead remained arduous and fraught with potential pitfalls, a fragile new hope was taking root. If we stayed the course through this harrowing inner excavation, perhaps we too could emerge renewed—like the Sword of Narsil from *The Lord of the Rings*, our fractured beings were reforged into something stronger and more whole than ever before.

While recovery was deeply uncomfortable at times, having space away from the demands of the world was crucial. It allowed me to begin building the tools and perspective necessary for a healthy, balanced life. Realizing I was in the right place was the wake-up call I needed.

As my time at Sierra Tucson drew to a close, I understood that the road to recognition was about more than acknowledging my struggles. It was about embracing the journey—with all its ups and downs—and finding strength in the community around me.

ADDICTION RECOVERY

was first introduced to addiction when I was fourteen years old. My older brother has courageously allowed me to share this story in the hope that it might help others struggling with addiction.

For months leading up to the discovery, my brother had been acting erratically, and I had no idea why. Then one day, he left his wallet in our shared bathroom. As I picked it up to move it away from the sink, a small tube fell out. Confused, I opened the wallet and found a tiny plastic bag filled with white powder.

I was stunned as the realization hit me—I was looking at cocaine, and it belonged to my brother.

Years earlier, at the start of high school, he'd fallen in with a group of so-called friends who experimented with alcohol and marijuana. Over time, he moved on to stronger substances—mushrooms, LSD, and eventually, cocaine. He had no idea how tightly these substances would grip his life.

After high school, his addiction worsened. But it wasn't until I found his stash that everything came to a head. I wrestled with the decision of whether I should say something. I didn't want to be a snitch—I knew the old saying, *snitches get stitches and end up in ditches*. I worried about how it might affect our relationship. But keeping his secret meant risking something far worse—losing him to an overdose or some other tragedy. That thought was unbearable, so I made my choice. I told my parents.

Soon after, my brother was checked into a rehab facility out of state to begin his recovery.

I'll never forget the pain and sorrow I felt watching him leave. We'd been close growing up, and losing him to addiction was heartbreaking. It took a toll on our entire family. Witnessing firsthand the devastation drugs and alcohol can cause, I made a vow—I would never touch alcohol or drugs, not even once. To this day, I've kept that promise.

After many difficult ups and downs, my brother eventually got clean and sober through a well-known twelve-step program. Having him free from the grip of addiction is a gift beyond measure. Thank you, big bro, for putting in the work to keep the demons at bay. When it was my turn to confront my own demons and face what lay ahead, your hard work and determination to break free became a powerful source of inspiration for me. I'm so grateful to still have you in my life, and I love you dearly.

ADDICTION: A DISEASE

It wasn't until many years later that I learned the dictionary defines a disease as "a disorder or abnormal condition that disrupts the normal functioning of the body or mind. It can be caused by infections, genetic factors, environmental influences, or lifestyle choices." How, then, does **addiction**[37] become a disease? Our brains are genetically wired with a survival list, a hierarchy of needs to keep us safe and alive, ordered from critically important at the top to less essential at the bottom. At the top are food, water, and shelter; lower down are job, relationships, hygiene, and personal integrity.

With an addiction—let's use meth as an example—the drug gradually moves up that survival list, pushing everything else down in priority. If I'm addicted to meth, getting it becomes more important than bathing or going to work. As I continue to use it, the addiction deepens, further entrenching the drug's priority over my relationships with my wife and kids. It keeps moving up the survival list. Eventually, meth becomes hardwired into my utmost survival instincts. It can become more vital than shelter or even food. I might find myself homeless, begging for handouts just to get my next fix. This shift in priorities, how it inserts itself and then climbs the survival list, is what makes addiction a disease; it takes control of us, much like the Cordyceps fungus in nature, known for turning ants into zombies—a concept often explored in horror movies.

I once heard an addict describe his brain as a Rolodex (some of my younger readers may need to Google that), with his emotions as cards. He couldn't control when he felt happy, sad, lost, or in control. He could only feel whatever emotion was on the card that came next in the stack. Often, he couldn't feel remorse for his actions until the "remorse card" came around again. The addiction completely controlled his emotions, with getting the next fix as the top priority.

This is why it's so hard for an addict to get clean: Because it isn't just about willpower or moral failing; it's a complex brain disease. To top it off, the emotions needed to rid oneself of the addiction only surface intermittently. Once an addict hits "rock bottom," as it's commonly called, the emotions necessary for recovery begin to emerge more frequently, motivating the addict to seek help.

The opioid crisis began in the late 1990s in the United States—characterized by mass addiction to opioids like prescription drugs, oxycodone, hydrocodone, codeine, and morphine—and continues to devastate communities today. A 2023 study in *JAMA Network Open* found that in 2021, only 1 in 5 adults in the U.S. dealing with opioid addiction got medication to help them recover. That means most people who need it aren't getting access to one of the best treatments out there. The study points out that making these meds easier to get could save a lot of lives by preventing overdoses.[38]

As a medical professional, I cannot stress enough how vital it is to approach addiction as a medical issue rather than a moral failing.

At Sierra Tucson, I watched in awe as my fellow warriors went through the rigors of getting clean from their substance abuse. Surprisingly, one of my fellow residents admitted that while quitting her substance abuse was terribly hard, the most challenging part of overcoming her addiction was facing all the pain and trauma she'd been numbing for years. She explained that it "felt like ripping off a bandage to reveal a festering wound underneath." Like this patient, at Sierra Tucson, I too confronted ugly truths about myself and my past that I'd been avoiding for years. It was excruciating but necessary, because you can't heal what you refuse to acknowledge.

Recovery is a daily choice, a constant recommitment to choose life over the siren song of addiction. Many have reported to me that some days, it feels impossibly hard, and the temptation to revert to old patterns is overwhelming. While I'm not going to even begin to compare my work addiction to some of the heartbreaking substance addictions I've seen, it's still been difficult for me to overcome. I drew so much satisfaction and fulfillment from my work, even though my addiction to it was crushing me.

To keep me from falling into old habits of biting off more than I can chew with work—and to help me decide what to pursue and what to leave behind—I follow Simon Sinek's advice on the Golden Circle. In his book *Start with Why*, he offers a structured way to assess your life's activities and understand your motivations. If I can't provide a detailed and honest answer about why I might start something that could awaken the workaholic monster, I let it go. Writing this book has been a journey of self-discovery, helping me clarify my "why." Why have I written this book? To help other Men Under Pressure find hope and healing. I truly hope that by sharing the hard-earned lessons my family and I have paid dearly for, my story will make a difference in someone's life. Take it from me: If you or someone you love is in the vice-like grip of addiction, there is hope! Recovery is possible. You can break free. It's hard but worth it—you are worth it!

MEN UNDER PRESSURE: GABE'S STORY

As I delved deeper into understanding addiction, I found other stories that highlight how addiction can take hold— not just through chemicals, but through the emotional turmoil that drives us to seek escape in the first place.

Let me tell you about my dear friend, whom I'll call "Gabe" for anonymity. Although he's given me full permission to share his story, we both agreed that changing his name was the best choice. I met Gabe at Sierra Tucson—he was my roommate and will always be my brother. Every day, we faced our own personal challenges in our therapeutic journeys, and our nightly recaps of what we learned and felt will always stay with me. I believe his unconditional love and kind encouragement helped unravel years of toxic shame. So thank you, Gabe, for being there for me. I consider my relationship with him one of the best things to come from my thirty-day stay at Sierra Tucson. Now, enough of the mushy stuff—let's get back to the matter at hand. Gabe's story is a rollercoaster ride—from the depths of addiction to the heights of recovery, a beacon of hope for anyone wrestling with their own demons.

Picture this: It's Staten Island, New York, in the late eighties and early nineties—not exactly a gay paradise, right? That's where Gabe grew up, realizing he was gay when he was around eleven years old. Talk about a recipe for angst. "I knew I liked boys at ten or eleven, probably around eleven, because that's when puberty started kicking in," Gabe told me, his voice tinged with humor and lingering pain.

Being gay in that time and place was as comfortable as a bed of nails. Gabe's brain tried to rationalize things: "I twisted my sexual orientation to make it okay. 'I'm not gay, just a little different.'" For a long time, denial convinced him it was something else entirely. But reality has a way of catching up. By high school, depression and suicidal thoughts became Gabe's unwelcome companions as he grappled with the fear that his parents would never accept him for being gay. When misery loves company, it throws a serious pity party.

Gabe's journey took him from college drinking to a hardcore addiction to mind-altering substances. We're talking heavy alcohol use in his twenties, cocaine in his early thirties, and eventually, the grand finale—crystal meth.

Gabe didn't simply decide one day to get better. It took a complete psychotic episode at work to kick him into gear as he hit "rock bottom." "One day, I overheard my boss talking about a compromising picture of me. Apparently, my neighbor took a photo of me smoking a crack pipe and sent it to them, and now they needed to fire me," Gabe recounted. (Spoiler alert: None of that actually happened. It was all in his meth-addled brain.)

Due to his daily meth use, he'd hallucinated the entire scenario. He was trapped in meth-induced psychosis, unable to distinguish fact from fiction, living in his own Matrix. He needed help, stat.

It turns out that sometimes, rock bottom is just the solid foundation you need to rebuild your life. Gabe found himself at Sierra Tucson, ready to face his demons head-on. And Sierra Tucson doesn't believe in half-measures; they threw everything but the kitchen sink at his addiction:

- EMDR
- Group and individual therapy
- CBT
- Mindfulness and breathing techniques

Post-rehab, Gabe maintained momentum with regular AA and Crystal Meth Anonymous meetings, even prioritizing sleep and exercise.

Now, drumroll, please...What were the results of all this hard work? Gabe achieved sobriety from meth. But it wasn't just about staying clean; his whole life did a 180.

He became more self-aware, better at managing his anxiety, and even shifted his career to the mental health field. Talk about turning lemons into lemonade!

Gabe's story is a testament to the resilience of the human spirit. Digging yourself out of a hole might involve a lot of therapy and more self-reflection than you ever thought possible, but it's worth it. As Gabe put it, "Shame loves the dark. Once you shine some light on it, you realize what you've been dreading isn't that big of a deal." Here's to bringing our shame into the light, facing our storms head-on, and coming out stronger than ever. Gabe did it, and so can you.

Listening to Gabe's struggles helped me recognize that my own pursuit of success was, in its own way, an addiction—one that kept me from addressing deeper issues. It was a wake-up call, prompting me to reflect on how I was living my life and what I needed to change.

"The opposite of addiction is not sobriety. The opposite of addiction is connection."

—JOHANN HARI

After answering the self-assessment questions in Appendix A, consider reflecting on your responses. Identifying patterns can be the first step toward understanding and addressing addiction. It may be beneficial to discuss these feelings and behaviors with a mental health professional for further support and guidance.

MEN UNDER PRESSURE: NICK'S STORY

Another powerful example of adaptability in the face of deep-seated struggles comes from Nick, whose journey through addiction led him down an unconventional path to recovery. His story highlights the importance of being open to different avenues of healing, even when they seem unconventional at first.

Over the years, I've encountered countless stories of struggle and triumph. But Nick's journey stands out vividly in my mind. I remember the day I decided to be vulnerable and opened up to him about my mental health struggles during lunch. He simply asked, "Whitney, how are you doing?" I could have given the typical response—"Awesome man, just living the dream. You?"—but something inside urged me to be honest. I felt comfortable saying, "I'm not well; I'm going through therapy and taking medication for my depression and anxiety." This sparked an incredible conversation. He encouraged me to share more, and I did. I felt nervous wondering if he would judge me or dismiss my struggles as weakness. Instead, he listened and revealed that he could relate, having faced difficult challenges himself.

Nick confessed that he'd struggled with a pornography addiction since he was just ten years old. While most kids were figuring out long division, Nick was tumbling down a digital rabbit hole that would haunt him for decades.

Pornography has a profound effect on the brain, particularly on pathways associated with pleasure and reward. When someone views porn, it triggers the release of dopamine, the chemical that makes us feel good. This response is similar to the effects of addictive substances, causing the brain to associate pornography with pleasure. Over time, this can lead to desensitization, where the brain becomes less responsive to the same level of stimulation. To achieve the same pleasurable feelings, a person might seek out more intense or extreme content. This repeated exposure can rewire the brain, prioritizing sexual imagery and affecting how someone responds to real-life relationships and experiences.

Additionally, regular use of pornography can impair emotional regulation, making it harder to find joy in everyday activities or connections with others. This rewiring can lead to compulsive behaviors, where individuals struggle to control their use of porn even when they recognize its negative impact on their lives. Understanding these effects highlights the challenges people face when trying to reduce or stop their pornography use, as the neural pathways created can generate a strong urge to continue.

Fast forward to adulthood: Nick had all the trappings of a picture-perfect life—a ring on his finger, a child running around the house, and a successful career. Yet his addiction clung to him like barnacles on a rusty ship. Like me, Nick hoped that life milestones would finally free him from the grip of porn, but it didn't happen. That pesky addiction persisted, leaving his mental health in shambles. Fortunately, Nick has an incredibly loving and supportive wife. Being honest with her about his struggles was critical for his healing. Her encouragement and understanding made all the difference. Instead of leaving him as he feared, she showed her love by not blowing up at him when he had slip-ups. They became a team, working together to tackle this issue. Nick explained that her unconditional support allowed him to explore various healing paths, but there was one in particular that made a significant difference: ayahuasca.

To Nick, every time he indulged in his vice of viewing pornography, he felt increasingly dirty and hopeless. Breaking that cycle was incredibly difficult, but not impossible. To him, traditional approaches—therapy, support groups, self-help books—felt inadequate, like bringing a squirt gun to a forest fire. Nick felt he needed something more potent and transformative.

That's when he discovered ayahuasca. Yes, that mind-bending brew that makes typical psychedelics look mild. Nick packed his bags and headed out of the United States for an ayahuasca retreat. Picture this: thirty to forty hungry souls huddled in sleeping bags under the stars while a shaman administered the ayahuasca and monitored its effects. After taking the drug, everyone fell asleep. Nick described his dreams as more vivid and real than anything he had ever experienced.

Now, while I can't fully endorse taking hallucinogens in the desert as a cure-all, Nick's experience was profound. He found himself on a psychedelic journey through his psyche, but it was no Disneyland adventure. He described being slowly lowered into a volcano filled with roiling, brown sludge that stank beyond description. I've watched a lot of movies, so I imagined it was like when the "heartless" acolyte gets sacrificed in the volcano in *Indiana Jones and the Temple of Doom*, but instead of lava, it was the Bog of Eternal Stench from the movie *Labyrinth*. The closer he got to that revolting sludge, the more repulsed he felt, recognizing it as a representation of pornography's toxic influence in his life.

When his body was finally submerged in the horrific sludge—*BAM*—he woke up, vomiting violently, as if auditioning for *The Exorcist*. But here's the twist: After this trippy, nightmare-puke experience, Nick felt the addiction lose its grip on him. It was as if his brain underwent a hard reboot, clearing away those addictive pathways.

Nick summed it up well when he said, "I knew I was vomiting that pornographic sludge out of me." Not exactly a Hallmark moment, but incredibly powerful. In time, he even returned for a second treatment—talk about commitment!

Nick's journey from digital pornographic sludge to freedom is a testament to the resilience of the human spirit. It reminds us that no matter how deep the hole is, there's always a way out—even if it involves a shaman, some hallucinations, and a whole lot of vomit.

So here's to Nick and to everyone fighting their own battles. Keep pushing, keep trying, and don't shy away from taking the road less traveled—just make sure it's legal first!

Nick's experience highlights the importance of celebrating every step forward, no matter how unconventional the path may be. Each moment of progress, whether marked by small victories or dramatic transformations, is worth acknowledging.

SIXTEEN

EMDR THERAPY

When I first settled onto the therapist's couch for my first experience with EMDR, a knot of anxiety twisted in my stomach. I tried to lighten the mood with a joke, but nothing came to mind—I was just too scared to think clearly, which was concerning.

This was my first appointment for EMDR, and I'd heard it was fantastic for healing inner demons, though I also knew it could be quite intense. My therapist exuded a tender, caring energy that immediately put me at ease. She introduced herself and gently asked me to share a bit about my life. "Well," I said, "I'm an orthodontist, married with three kids, and I'm pretty messed up." She laughed and replied, "Aren't we all?"

Despite her kind demeanor, I quickly realized that getting well wouldn't involve a few cushy therapy sessions over herbal tea and hugs. This was going to be hard work.

Sierra Tucson embraced a vigorous philosophy: a full-frontal assault on the demons and traumas poisoning my psyche. It would be the hardest work of my life, but I'd come to Sierra as a broken man, my mind and spirit in disarray. I was ready—desperate, even—to place myself completely in their care and endure whatever challenging treatments they prescribed. The pain of remaining shackled by my inner demons had finally outweighed the pain of pursuing freedom, no matter how excruciating that journey might be.

In truth? EMDR would turn out to be my ayahuasca.

EMDR AND ME

EMDR turned out to be one of the most powerful and viscerally exhausting experiences of my life.

I'll never forget how my therapist described it: "Think of it this way, Whitney. Our brains naturally process life experiences and file them away. When we experience something, our brains flood with information that travels back and forth across the midline that separates the left and right sides of your brain. Once this information crosses back and forth several times, the brain processes it into a memory and files it away. But with particularly traumatic events, as a way of protecting us, the information processing system in our brains can get bypassed.

"If the mind fully processes something too traumatic for it to safely handle, it can result in the entire brain shutting down, causing the person to go into shock and 'freezing in place' when instead they need to flee. It is part of the body's fight-or-flight mechanism. In order to bypass the harmful 'freeze' state, and in hopes of keeping us alive, the brain takes the 'unsafe' traumatic information—along with the memories, associated feelings, and physical sensations—and locks them away in an unprocessed state deep in our psyche like little trauma nuggets that are too difficult to process and keep you safe at the same time. EMDR helps jiggle those stubborn trauma nuggets loose so your brain can finally process and integrate them."

If you've ever had something stuck in your kitchen sink garbage disposal, like a peach pit, you know you have to reach in to pull it out before it ruins the machine. It's messy and sometimes scary, but it's necessary for the system to function effectively. These stuck trauma nuggets live in our brains and, if left untreated, will manifest as anxiety, depression, addiction, and other mental issues. EMDR gets those trauma nuggets out and fills their voids with helpful and positive memories.

Fascinated by the science behind this process, I wondered if EMDR could really help me overcome the traumas that had haunted me for so long. There was only one way to find out. Over the following weeks, I diligently went through the EMDR protocol with my therapist at Sierra Tucson. The initial sessions focused on my history and identifying the specific traumatic memories we would target. Just verbalizing some of those experiences released emotions I had bottled up for years. We also delved into inner-child work. If you'd told me there was an inner child in me struggling with feeling safe and that his emotions affected my own, I would have laughed. But after learning about it and experiencing it firsthand, I can honestly say that inner-child work is transformative.

During the reprocessing phases, my therapist had me bring up traumatic memories in vivid detail while watching a light move left and right on a light bar in front of me. My head remained still; only my eyes moved back and forth. To ramp it up, she had me hold buzzers in my hands that buzzed in sync with the moving light. Finally, for maximum effectiveness, she put headphones on me that beeped in one ear as the light hit the end of the bar. I was experiencing simultaneous visual, auditory, and tactile stimulation, designed to alternately activate both sides of my brain and dislodge the deeply buried trauma lingering in my mind. The bilateral stimulation helps the brain reprocess stuck memories, allowing them to cross the midline and get processed properly. With the moving lights, humming buzzers, and beeping headphones, the intensity had been turned up to eleven.

At first, it felt strange to shift between recounting painful experiences and the rapid eye movements. But after a few sets, something started to change. The memory itself began to lose its charge, the sharp sting fading into a dull ache. Waves of emotion would wash over me, only to ebb away just as quickly.

With each session, we dug deeper into the roots of my trauma—self-loathing beliefs, visceral bodily sensations tied to past events. Each time, EMDR's desensitization process seemed to unravel another knotted thread in my psyche.

There were breakthroughs where long-suppressed memories bubbled up unexpectedly, unlocking doors I didn't even know existed in my mind. Other times, I emerged from a session feeling utterly drained, as if my soul had been wrung dry. My therapist reassured me this was all part of the process, emotional housekeeping to clear out the psychic debris. As a first responder and veterans' PTSD specialist, she often witnessed grown men crying as the pent-up pain and fear from past traumas were finally released. "I've seen men in here who could bench press a Volkswagen balling like babies," she said. Through these last several years, I've learned that crying is normal—it's part of the healing process. When your body is injured, blood comes out. When your soul and psyche are injured, tears come out.

It was one of the most harrowing yet strangely healing experiences of my life. I can't say the process was ever easy or comfortable, but working through those stuck traumas, giving them a way to be metabolized and integrated, brought an incredible lightness. It felt like releasing shackles I'd bound myself with for decades without realizing it.

I can discuss my past traumas so matter-of-factly because of the miraculous healing effects of EMDR. Previously, just thinking about what happened would send me into a tailspin. Now, it's merely a blip on my journey in this lifelong adventure of seeking peace and happiness. I highly recommend the book *Getting Past Your Past: Take Control of Your Life With Self-Help Techniques from EMDR Therapy* by Dr. Francine Shapiro, the amazing psychologist who discovered and developed EMDR therapy.

MEN UNDER PRESSURE: TYLER'S STORY

Tyler Andrus, a licensed therapist, also has had a trans-formational journey through EMDR therapy that has not only transformed his personal life but also revolution-ized his professional practice. Sometimes, the teacher becomes the student, the doctor becomes the patient, and the therapist finds himself on the couch.

I first crossed paths with Tyler in church, long before either of us could have predicted the parallel journeys we'd embark upon. Years later, our stories intertwined again, bound by the thread of EMDR. Tyler, a specialist in EMDR, found himself caught in a cruel irony: He was the healer in need of healing, the guide lost in his own maze.

Growing up, Tyler watched several close family mem-bers struggle with overwhelming health and financial challenges. These traumatic experiences lodged in his mind, creating a mental cascade that made him feel doomed to repeat their struggles. Faced with a life that felt like an unending series of crises, he decided to con-front it head-on, signing up for things he knew he would hate—digging those traumatic shards out of his psyche once and for all. "I sign up for the crappy things I know I'm gonna hate because in the end, I know I'll love the results," he confessed, his self-deprecating humor barely masking the underlying pain.

This tendency to intentionally choose difficult and

possibly detrimental situations led Tyler into a work environment that was slowly grinding him down. Stress, self-doubt, and anxiety became his constant companions.

Bravely, Tyler decided to enter the one place he feared most: his own psyche. He dove into EMDR therapy, the very technique he practiced, with the desperation of a man drowning in unresolved traumas.

He explained to me, "Imagine EMDR as a mental Heimlich maneuver for trauma. It helps dislodge those sticky, painful memories lodged in our brains, preventing proper processing. Through guided eye movements (or sometimes taps or tones), EMDR helps the brain reprocess these traumatic memories, taking the sting out of them."

As Tyler went through his EMDR sessions, he faced the ghosts of his past. It was subtle at first, but with each session, each confrontation with his buried traumas, he felt a shift. Amid this internal excavation, Tyler had an epiphany about his work situation. "Instead of working harder, let's work smarter. Let's do something professionally that truly honors my energy and overall needs," he realized. This simple yet profound insight led him to make a bold move—starting his own private practice. It was a leap of faith that allowed him to create a working environment aligned with his newfound insights and healing. He was no longer trapped in a cycle of choosing difficult situations at work that didn't align with his life goals.

With his confidence growing, Tyler began connecting with clients on a deeper level. His own experiences of vulnerability and healing through EMDR formed a bridge of empathy. "There's no way I'd have been able to start my own practice without EMDR. I'd still be stuck where I was a few years ago," Tyler shared, his voice filled with gratitude and awe.

The most profound change, however, was in Tyler's relationship with himself. Patterns of self-sabotage began to fade, replaced by a growing sense of self-compassion and understanding.

His journey is a powerful reminder of the importance of self-care in the helping professions. It's easy to fall into the trap of thinking that because we help others, we don't need help ourselves. As Tyler's story shows, sometimes the best thing a healer can do is become the patient.

Tyler's story is not just a testament to the power of EMDR; it's also a reminder of the courage it takes to face our inner struggles. It highlights the strength found in vulnerability and the healing that comes when we dare to confront the parts of ourselves we'd rather keep hidden.

Tyler's journey from struggling therapist to confident practitioner beautifully illustrates the ripple effect of personal healing. By confronting his own demons, he not only transformed his life but also enhanced his ability to guide others through their darkest hours.

MEN UNDER PRESSURE: CHARLES'S STORY

As a law enforcement officer, Charles had seen some of the darkest aspects of humanity—the violence, the despair, the senseless loss of life. I can still picture the look on his face as he described the countless times he walked into an opioid house and had to step around over-dosed people. I can't even begin to fathom the trauma of repeatedly finding lifeless bodies strewn across the floor—and not all of them were adults.

But he told me that it wasn't until he nearly lost his own life that he truly understood the depths of the epidemic he was fighting.

It happened after a routine drug bust. Charles and his team had seized a large quantity of narcotics, including fentanyl—a synthetic opioid fifty times more potent than heroin. As he drove back to the station with the drugs in his car, he suddenly felt dizzy and short of breath. At first, he dismissed it as stress—the long hours, the constant exposure to danger. But as the minutes passed, he realized something was seriously wrong.

Unbeknownst to him, the fentanyl had leaked from its packaging, releasing deadly fumes into his vehicle. He passed out behind the wheel, veered off the road, and crashed into a ditch.

Fortunately, an officer following behind him recognized the signs of an overdose. Pulling Charles from the vehicle, they found his breathing dangerously slow, his skin turning a sickly shade of blue. Without hesitation, his fellow officers administered Narcan and performed CPR.

If not for their quick actions, Charles might not have survived.

But the near-death experience was just the beginning of Charles's journey. In the weeks and months that followed, he found himself plagued by nightmares, flashbacks, and a constant sense of dread. He was jumpy and irritable, lashing out at his loved ones and struggling to find joy in the things that used to bring him happiness. It wasn't until he sought help from a therapist specializing in PTSD that he began to understand the toll that the years of trauma had taken on his mind and body.

Through a combination of EMDR therapy, medication, and peer support, Charles slowly began to heal. He learned coping strategies for managing his symptoms, and he found solace in connecting with other first responders who had experienced similar traumas. And as he began to share his story with others, he realized that he had the power to make a difference, to help others who might be struggling with the same demons that had nearly destroyed him.

Today, Charles has retired after a lifelong successful career in law enforcement. And while the scars of his trauma may never fully fade, he's learned to wear them as a badge of honor, a reminder of the incredible resilience and strength that lies within him.

While I was at Sierra Tucson, hearing him speak about his experiences with such raw honesty and vulnerability was truly inspiring. And if there's one thing I've learned from Charles's story, it's that hope can be found in even the darkest of places. When we have the courage to share our stories and connect with others, we have the power to change lives, one day at a time.

Charles's journey, like so many others, teaches us that the strength to keep fighting often comes from the connections we forge and the stories we share. These narratives of resilience are not just about survival—they are about thriving despite the odds, and they remind us that every step forward is a testament to the courage within us all.

"It always seems impossible until it's done."
—NELSON MANDELA

SEVENTEEN

THE ROLE OF INNER-CHILD WORK

EMDR unraveled the tangled threads of trauma in my mind, but deeper wounds still needed tending. That's where inner-child work came in, offering a path to reconnect with the most vulnerable parts of myself.

Before heading to Sierra Tucson, if someone had told me that a significant portion of my issues stemmed from an injured inner child, I would have dismissed them. Now, I'm a firm believer in the power of this technique. Inner-child therapy involves nurturing the part of myself that embodies childhood experiences, emotions, and beliefs that continue to influence my adult life. By engaging in this work, I aimed to address the roots of my trauma and cultivate a more compassionate relationship with myself.

Inner-child therapy focuses on healing emotional wounds from our childhood. We all have a "child" inside us, representing our younger selves and the experiences that shaped our thoughts, feelings, and behaviors as adults, often in ways we might not realize. Inner-child therapy encourages you to reconnect with your younger self, acknowledging the feelings and needs that may have been neglected or hurt in the past. This can involve exploring memories, expressing emotions, and visualizing nurturing that inner child. Through this process, you can work through unresolved issues, develop self-compassion, and learn healthier ways to cope with adult challenges. Ultimately, inner-child therapy fosters healing and promotes a more positive relationship with yourself.

One of the most pivotal moments of my journey at Sierra involved delving into those primal childhood wounds. My therapist guided me through visualization exercises to connect with the scared little boy still trapped inside me. The goal was to offer him the nurturing, protection, and unconditional love he needed to feel safe again. Essentially, I, as the grown-up version of Whitney, was in control of our lives and capable of caring for both the adult Whitney and the young Whitney filled with fear and uncertainty.

The process began with writing a letter to my younger self—a daunting task. My group therapist asked me to write to eight-year-old Whitney, detailing the hard and terrible things that would happen to him as he grew up, including experiences of abuse, feelings of invisibility and worthlessness, and painful betrayals that would affect him for years. I had to confront all the raw hurts, fears, and existential terrors that little Whitney faced. As I filled the tear-stained pages with my anguished scrawl, I felt that small, fragile part of myself trembling within. Writing those pages was incredibly difficult, but the next part would prove to be even more challenging.

The following day in a group therapy session mostly composed of women, two chairs were placed facing each other. I would sit in one, and the other would remain empty, reserved for Little Whitney. I read the letter aloud to him. It was one of the most embarrassing, vulnerable, gut-wrenching experiences of my life. Struggling to read through my tears, I shared what awaited that sweet, innocent boy. Flashes of memory emerged, dissolving into waves of repressed anger, sadness, and pain, leading me to purge with wracking sobs. When I finally finished reading the letter—after what felt like forever—my pent-up rage came rushing out, and it wasn't pretty. My whole body began to shake as adrenaline flooded my bloodstream. My eyes began darting all around the room, hunting for an unseen threat. It was when my therapist saw my fists clench and my body tensing for a fight that he stepped in. He asked me to push my fist against his palm to start venting the rage. Soon, overpowering him, he handed me a pillow and told me to try to rip it in half. Even more rage erupted out of me.

Finally, my therapist encouraged me to push against the wall of the room with all of my strength. As I physically embodied the wrath consuming me—pouring all my strength into pushing against the wall—the room felt as though it was shaking as the pictures on the wall rattled and the clock fell from the wall as I yelled in absolute blinding rage. After the rage subsided, I felt utterly spent, a hollow shell of a man. I slumped against the wall, crying, and my therapist helped me up, where I received hugs and support from my incredibly compassionate group. The final step of the inner-child healing process was to burn the letter I'd written to Little Whitney, signifying that it was finally over.

The entire process was grotesquely uncomfortable yet profoundly cathartic. Going back and rewriting my childhood narrative from a place of wholeness let my inner child know he was finally seen, heard, loved, and protected as he always deserved to be. More than five years have passed since that therapeutic experience, and my inner child still feels safe and secure.

Through this journey, I gained insight into how my early experiences shaped my self-image, relationships, and coping mechanisms. I recognized that the negative beliefs and patterns I developed in response to childhood trauma no longer served me; they were holding me back from a fulfilling life. By providing my inner child with the love, validation, and support that I lacked in my past, I began to release emotional burdens and develop healthier ways of relating to myself and others. I learned to challenge limiting beliefs, set boundaries, and prioritize self-care— all essential components of my ongoing healing journey.

After experiencing the transformative effects of self-care work at Sierra Tucson, I recognized the importance of continuing this practice in my daily life. Healing is an ongoing process, and nurturing my wounded self would be a lifelong commitment.

To incorporate self-care into my routine, I developed practices and rituals that keep me connected to my current self and my inner child, providing the support and validation needed for continued growth and healing. These practices include journaling, meditation, and other forms of self-reflection.

I also value maintaining an ongoing dialogue with myself and my inner child. By regularly checking in with my emotions, needs, and desires, I build a stronger, more compassionate relationship with myself. This dialogue involves speaking to my inner child directly, writing letters, and engaging in creative activities that allow for self-expression, such as coloring with colored pencils. There's something deeply calming about pulling out my tin of Prismacolor colored pencils, sharpening each one slowly, inhaling the scent of freshly cut wood, and honing them to a fine point. I have various mandala coloring books that help me zone out and enter a flow state. When all I have to do is choose colors and stay within the lines, my brain hits a reset button, relieving my worries and fears.

Additionally, I learned a fascinating technique to uncover subconscious thoughts: By writing a question with my dominant hand and the answer with my nondominant hand, I allow my subconscious mind to express itself freely—even if the penmanship is terrible.

Throughout this ongoing process, I sought support from therapists and counselors. Having a safe space to share experiences, process emotions, and receive guidance from others on similar paths has been crucial for my continued growth and healing.

Working with my inner child opened up a new understanding of myself, but the journey didn't end there. Only through consistent self-care and introspection did I begin to truly transform my self-perception and healing journey.

> "To be happy is to be able to become aware
> of your inner child and to listen to it."
> —PAULO COELHO

MEN UNDER PRESSURE: DOUG'S STORY

I met Doug after Sierra Tucson, and his story broke my heart. Doug grew up in a troubled home that eventually ended with both parents going to jail for drug dealing. As a young teen, it only got worse—he ended up in the care of a relative who introduced him to sexually suggestive material, which then sadly led to sexual abuse.

Doug shared with me that he felt powerless in that situation. This was the one adult who was supposed to protect and care for him, yet instead, he was the one sexually abusing him.

Tragically, when a child is abused by an adult caretaker, they are often wedged between a rock and a hard place. On one hand, if they report the abuse, they'll lose the support and caretaking of the adult; on the other hand, they hate themselves for not taking steps to stop the abuse from happening and are filled with anger at their abuser.

Repressing this anger causes something terrible to happen inside the child. The fear and anger they feel gets pushed down and internalized because they don't dare direct it at their abusive caregiver—that would only make things worse. That anger and fear then switch internally to guilt and shame. The victim feels ashamed for allowing this to happen to them and tries to hide it from the world. The shame that is created can be even more insidious than the abuse itself. It will tell the victim that they deserved to be abused, that they are worthless and will always be worthless, that they are subhuman.

This is how shame turns toxic, and it will permeate throughout every aspect of the victim's life. This toxic shame will ultimately lead to feelings of depression, anxiety, and overall worthlessness, which oftentimes lead to self-destructive behaviors and addiction.

Doug, now a drug- and sex-addicted adult, knew he needed help with his quickly deteriorating mental health, but he couldn't pin down what was ultimately causing his depression. After spending quality time with his therapist, Doug finally did something he'd never done in his entire life—he told his therapist that he'd been abused as a child.

He told me how hot tears and wracking sobs exploded out of him in a wave of fear, horror, and shame. He explained that once he finally let that poisonous secret out, he was shaking so badly he thought he would fall off of the couch. His whole life, he'd been terrified of anyone finding out due to that toxic guilt and shame that so frequently happens to victims of abuse.

The guilt and shame doesn't only happen with sexual abuse; it can manifest with physical, mental, and emotional abuse, too. If a child is abused and repeatedly feels angry or afraid of a caregiver, more often than not, that anger and fear will turn to guilt and shame.

It was only after earning Doug's trust that the therapist could gently coax the truth from him, but once Doug had spoken the horrific words out loud, he immediately started to feel better. That terrible shame, which hides in the dark recesses of our minds, feeding on our fear and guilt, dies kicking and screaming once we drag it into the light. Doug was well on his way to ultimately healing that inner child, who was so savagely abused by a trusted caretaker who took advantage of Doug's pain after losing his parents to lives of crime.

Like Doug, anyone who has experienced childhood trauma carries buried shards that need healing. Once his inner child felt safe and secure, Doug was able to continue on his healing journey. Sometimes, the things that hold us back long to be set free; they yearn for acknowledgment before they can be released.

If you have a "terrible secret" that you're hiding from the world, it's likely that you're grappling with traumatic experiences that undermine your sense of peace and safety. Your inner child may still be terrified of what happened all those years ago.

Take the time to explore your feelings and secrets. It might be the perfect moment to seek out a therapist and let go of the pain once and for all.

CONCLUSION

My healing journey involved a combination of different therapeutic approaches, each targeting specific aspects of my trauma and recovery. EMDR and inner-child work both played crucial roles in my healing process, working together to address the complex nature of my trauma.

EMDR helped me to process and integrate traumatic memories, reducing their emotional intensity and allowing me to develop a more coherent narrative of my experiences. By reducing the distress associated with these memories, it helped create a more stable foundation for the other therapeutic work I was engaged in.

Inner-child work addressed the relational and developmental impacts of my early experiences, helping me to repair myself and develop a more nurturing and compassionate relationship with my own emotions and needs.

Over the years, I've come to recognize the nonlinear nature of healing, with progress often involving a complex interplay of different therapeutic modalities and ongoing self-work. By embracing a holistic approach and remaining committed to my own growth and recovery, I was able to navigate the challenges of healing complex trauma and emerge with a greater sense of wholeness and resilience.

I've also recognized that the more self-compassion I'm able to show myself, the happier I am. When I turn into my own constructive coach versus a disgruntled critic, I feel and do much better. The negative self-talk melts away, and I begin to love myself more. There's a famous scripture in the Bible that says, "Love thy neighbor as thyself." When I think about this verse, I wonder what it means to love myself. I believe it means taking care of myself like I would my neighbor. I wouldn't tear down or belittle my neighbor, so why would I do that to myself? I would do what I could to help a neighbor, and thus in turn, I can do more to help myself feel better and succeed in my endeavors.

I had faced my demons, swam in the blackest waters of my psyche, and come out the other side reborn. The path ahead would never be perfect, but at least I could walk it unburdened by the weights that had nearly dragged me under before. I was finally free.

COMING HOME

As I readied myself to depart Sierra Tucson, I felt an unexpected pang of sadness at leaving. So much anguish expunged, so much darkness transformed into hard-won light and integration.

As I was dragging my suitcases down the hall on my way home, I caught a glimpse of myself in the hallway mirror and had to smile at the man looking back at me. Still a bit wan and rough around the edges, sure, but also emanating a quiet soulfulness—the unmistakable patina of someone who has stared into the abyss and come out the other side, forever marked by the descent but now armed with the battle visors of hard-earned wisdom and resilience. I faced my fears, pushed through the shadows, and found inexplicable light and expansiveness on the other side. I reclaimed my life.

As I walked toward my car in the parking lot, I felt a surge of gratitude for the champions—both the professionals and the loved ones—who had fought for me to make this transformation possible. Though this sojourn of healing was hardly "complete," I knew the blessings of this interim awakening would reverberate through every aspect of my existence from here on out. As I slowly drove out of the parking lot, I saw the sign that sits at the entrance. When you enter Sierra Tucson, the sign outside reads, "Expect a Miracle." I remember reading that sign the day of my arrival and hoping and praying I would receive a miracle, a miracle of healing. Now that I was leaving the parking lot, I saw to my surprise that the back of the sign read, "You Are the Miracle." I choked up a little bit realizing that I'd found my self-worth and had let go of the toxic shame that had been holding me back for years. I had indeed received a miracle. I got Whitney back! The path was fresher now, my step was lighter, and my heart was reopened to the possibilities of what lay ahead.

My time at Sierra Tucson was marked by these profound therapies—each one peeling back layers of pain and revealing a more resilient self underneath. As I finally drove away, I knew the road ahead would be challenging, but I was finally ready to face it.

I was ready to greet the world anew.

> "What lies behind us and what
> lies before us are tiny matters
> compared to what lies within us."
> —RALPH WALDO EMERSON

A NEW WHITNEY

Throughout my stay at Sierra Tucson, I was both excited and terrified of the day I'd go home. I was eager to reunite with Margaret and the kids, but I knew the real challenge lay ahead in adapting to my new life. I desperately wanted to demonstrate to my family that "happy and healthy" Whitney was back, so I planned a surprise homecoming, returning a day earlier than scheduled from Sierra Tucson. The excitement of my doctors and therapists who supported me in this plan bolstered my confidence, and the emotional farewell from Sierra Tucson marked a significant milestone in my journey.

The drive home was a mix of emotions, with "Here Comes the Sun" by The Beatles blasting through the speakers on repeat, symbolizing hope and renewal. I pulled into the garage, parked, and quietly snuck into the house. Margaret was busy with one of her projects, unaware of my early return. Standing in the doorway, I called out, "Hey, Girlie, I'm home!"

Margaret froze, her body tense with shock at hearing my voice. Slowly turning around, she exclaimed, "You're not supposed to be home until tomorrow!" Her face flashed through a range of emotions as she processed the unexpected surprise. I stood there smiling, arms outstretched, waiting for her reaction. As the initial surprise faded, the reality of our reunion began to sink in. Finally, she overcame the initial shock and ran into my arms, both of us crying as we held each other tightly. After some kisses and playful banter, she punched my arm and said, "You scared me sneaking in like that!"

But I could tell by the way she held me tight, how she breathed me in deeply with her head on my chest, that she was ready to accept the new Whitney. She could feel that the man I once was, confident and strong, was back. I felt the fears and worries she'd been carrying for the last month melt away as I told her I loved her and how I felt like me again. I thanked her for her incredible support and for running the show as I went away for thirty long days.

As she looked up into my eyes to see if I truly believed what I was saying to her, she saw my determination and desire to be the best husband and father I could be. I'd gone into Sierra Tucson broken and scarred, and through the searing forge of healing, I came out shiny and new. I made a promise to her and myself right then that I would never again drive myself into such dire straits. Now I knew what I knew, and like Maya Angelou said, "I did what I knew...and when I knew better, I did better." I was going to do better from here on out.

Next, it was time to surprise the kids! They were at school and would be arriving home at different times. I set up one of my classic Dad tricks: a sticky-note scavenger hunt.

I placed the first note on the front door saying, "Check the playroom," in my handwriting. When my daughters got off the school bus together, they burst through the front door yelling, "Dad?! Daddy, are you here?" They dashed through the house room by room, following the clues I'd left, as their excitement and anticipation grew. The last note directed them to "check the couch," which I'd been hiding behind when they first entered. They came running down the stairs, winded from their frantic search, and found me sitting on the couch with a huge smile on my face and my arms outstretched wide.

Their faces lit up with joy, and they squealed with delight as they dove into my arms, showering me with kisses and giggles. I hugged and tickled them as we laughed and cried together on the couch for what felt like an eternity of pure bliss.

Then, with the help of my newly recruited prankster daughters, we prepared to surprise our third and oldest child, my son. The girls helped me reset the sticky notes before hiding behind the couch with me. Arriving home from school, my son started his own scavenger hunt, running through the house until he found me. I could tell he was getting more and more frantic to find me, his voice calling out, "Dad?! Dad, are you really home?"

When he found me on the couch waiting for him, with the girls watching from another part of the room, he launched himself into my arms, breaking down in tears, pleading, "Please don't ever leave me again, Dad." I reassured him, "Never again, son, never again." It was one of the most tender moments of my life, knowing I'd restored my relationship with my sweet family. As we laughed and hugged, the full impact of my return began to take hold. They'd endured a month of uncertainty and dread. Will our husband and father be able to recover from his mental breakdown and continue to do his part in leading our household? Absolutely I will.

This homecoming was more than just a reunion; it was a testament to my commitment to maintaining the progress I'd made. The therapy and growth I experienced at Sierra Tucson had transformed my traumatic past into just that—a part of my past. I was ready to move forward, leaving behind the poison that once plagued my mind and body, and embrace a future filled with hope and healing.

But the journey didn't end with my return home. The real work was just beginning.

> **"Family is not an important thing.**
> **It's everything."**
> —MICHAEL J. FOX

LASTING LIFESTYLE CHANGES

Sierra Tucson's staff emphasized the importance of lasting lifestyle changes, comparing inpatient treatment to training wheels. This analogy resonated with me because it underscored that the real test of my recovery would begin once I left the supportive environment of the facility. I envisioned myself transforming into a new man, filled with zen-like calm, meditating at sunrise, practicing yoga, and journaling daily. I imagined living a life of balance, serenity, and self-care, fully committed to these new habits. Well, those grand plans of morning meditation and greeting the sun in a glorious way didn't quite unfold as I'd hoped.

The hardest part of recovery was putting into practice the healthy coping skills I'd learned at Sierra Tucson. In the structured and supportive environment of the treatment center, it was easier to maintain new habits. But outside, amid the chaos and triggers of everyday life, it became a challenge. I quickly realized that embracing my "new normal" would be a process rather than an instant transformation. This journey involved setbacks, self-doubt, and resisting the urge to slip back into old, unhealthy coping mechanisms.

Sierra Tucson had dragged my demons into the daylight, where I could finally confront them. In the grand scheme of things, was twenty minutes of daily meditation or resisting the siren call of sixty-hour work weeks really a Herculean feat? All I needed was to keep showing up for myself, one small victory at a time.

Fortunately, my Sierra Tucson team equipped me with an arsenal of transformative techniques to navigate the uneven terrain of recovery. From meditation—mainly slow and controlled breathwork—to journaling and healthy communication, I now had an array of tools to excavate my authentic self from the rubble: meditation, journaling, spending time outdoors, cold exposure, prayer and spirituality, ongoing therapy, and engaging in hobbies. The challenge was remembering to actually use them instead of defaulting to my trusty old coping mechanisms (read: work binges and emotional hibernation).

But I've done it, and I'll keep doing it. I'm committed, for my family and for myself. And, because you're reading this right now, for you, too—to serve as continued proof that healing is possible. Thank you for helping to drive me forward. I'm here to return the favor. You have my word.

SHARE YOUR STORY AND INSPIRE OTHERS

YOUR VOICE MATTERS.

If *Men Under Pressure* helped you, your story could help another man take the first step toward healing.

Leave a review on Amazon:
Your review helps others find this book—just a few words can make a big difference. Scan the QR code or visit *review.menunderpressure.com*.

YOUR STORY CAN INSPIRE OTHERS.

I'd love to hear how this book has impacted you. Whether it's a shift in mindset, a new habit, or a major breakthrough—your experience could show another man what's possible.

Submit your success story here:
Scan the QR code or visit
success.menunderpressure.com.

Thank you for being part of this movement.
Let's keep breaking the silence—together.

AFTERWORD

I'm happy to share that Risas Dental and Braces, the dental company I helped start, continues to thrive. Over the years, we've faced our fair share of challenges, but through it all, we've stayed true to our mission of providing high-quality, affordable dental care to those who need it most. I couldn't be prouder of the incredible team we've built and the positive impact we've had on our community.

After five long years of panic attacks at the mere thought of treating patients, I finally took a significant step—I saw patients for the first time without having a panic attack. It was a milestone that filled me with both relief and gratitude. However, will I return to the clinic full-time? No, that chapter of my life has closed.

While my symptoms aren't as severe as they once were, I still experience PTSD related to the clinic and seeing patients. I've learned not to tempt fate and risk undoing the progress I've worked so hard to achieve. My psychiatrist, Dr. Saba Monsoor, put it into perspective when she said, "Whitney, you have PTSD. You cannot immerse yourself in your traumatic experiences once a week and expect to come out unscathed. Imagine a soldier being asked to return to the front lines just once a week while suffering from PTSD. It would destroy them, and it will ultimately destroy you."

That said, there's a big difference between saying, "I can't do orthodontics," and "I am choosing not to do orthodontics." For me, this choice is about prioritizing my mental health and well-being.

Even though I'm no longer in the clinic, I remain committed to advocating for mental health. My focus is on helping others find hope and healing, just as I have.

As much as I love my work with Risas, I've also been learning important lessons about the power of boundaries in my personal life. As someone who has always been a people pleaser and an overachieving workaholic, saying "no" or putting my own needs first isn't always easy. But over the past few years, I've come to realize how critical it is to set clear boundaries and stick to them, even when it feels uncomfortable or difficult.

Setting boundaries may seem rude to others, but it's actually an act of kindness. By being honest about what I'm comfortable doing, I become more authentic, and my anxiety decreases. My ability to say no improves, and my well-being is protected.

Of course, that's easier said than done. There have been plenty of times when my boundaries have been tested—whether it's a friend asking for a favor I can't realistically commit to or a business associate wanting me to take on more than I can handle. In those moments, it's all too easy to fall back into old patterns of overextending myself or sacrificing my own well-being for the sake of others.

Here's the thing: Every time I've let my boundaries slip, I've paid the price. Whether it's burnout, resentment, or a general sense of being overwhelmed, the consequences of not standing up for myself are always more painful than the temporary discomfort of saying no.

That's why I've been working hard to get better at setting and enforcing my boundaries in both my personal and professional life. It isn't always easy. There are times when I still struggle with guilt or the fear of disappointing others. But I'm learning to reframe those feelings, reminding myself that setting boundaries isn't selfish or unkind; it's a necessary act of self-care and self-respect.

THE SUPPORT OF MY FAMILY AND FRIENDS

I couldn't do any of this without the support of my amazing wife, Margaret. For more than twenty-two years, she's been my rock and my voice of reason when I get lost in the weeds of people-pleasing and overcommitment. When I do slip up and let my boundaries slide, she gently reminds me of what's important, encouraging me to put myself first and trust that the world will keep spinning even if I say no every once in a while.

Another silver lining in all this mental health work is that my kids are now comfortable talking about their emotional well-being, both when they're doing well and when they're not. Knowing that we, as parents, have fostered an environment where it's okay to "not be okay" feels incredible. There have even been instances when our children recognized toxic behaviors in their friends and used their own boundaries to protect themselves.

My friends and family have been incredibly supportive throughout this journey. They continue to check in on me, ensuring I'm doing well. Knowing I have a history of burying my issues under a comedic façade, they take the time to ask how I'm doing in more personal settings, giving me the opportunity to open up if needed. I especially want to emphasize that I don't harbor blame or resentment toward my parents for the abuse I experienced in my childhood. That blame rests on my abuser. I've had many meaningful conversations with my mom and dad about the past, and they understand that I love them deeply and am incredibly grateful for their support in my life.

TAKE CARE OF YOURSELF FIRST

So that's where I'm at these days—still learning, growing, and figuring out how to navigate the tricky waters of boundary-setting and self-care. Through it all, I'm reminded of the incredible power of hope and resilience, not just in overcoming addiction and trauma, but in all areas of life. Because at the end of the day, that's what setting boundaries is all about—it's about having the courage to stand up for ourselves, to believe in our own worth and value, and to trust that by taking care of ourselves first, we can show up more fully and authentically for the people and causes we care about most.

If there's one thing I've learned on this wild journey, it's that hope and resilience aren't just feel-good buzzwords—they're the foundation of a life well-lived. They give us the strength to keep going when things get tough, to pick ourselves up when we fall, and to believe in the possibility of a brighter tomorrow, even in the darkest of times.

I'd like you to think back to the Introduction of this book:

There I was, thirty-six years old, hyperventilating, drenched in sweat, alternating between vomiting into the toilet and curling up in the fetal position on the cold floor of the restroom of my orthodontic office. I was in the throes of a severe panic attack, and it wasn't my first. My mental health had been unraveling for some time, but I kept telling myself that a "real man" doesn't show weakness. He doesn't show fear. He's supposed to be the immovable pillar of strength, the rock that others rely on in life's storm.

Now, here I am, forty-four years old: calm, collected, free of anxiety and depression, hormonally balanced, living honestly, and free of toxic shame. As I reflect on this journey, I face the questions that once haunted me as I hit rock bottom.

HOW DID I END UP HERE?

By not taking care of myself. I had ignored my needs for so long that I allowed myself to fall into disrepair.

WHAT COULD I HAVE DONE DIFFERENTLY?

I could have recognized the red flags in my life and taken a personal inventory of how I was truly feeling. I'd hidden from my emotions for years, burying them beneath the responsibilities of work, fatherhood, and maintaining my ego. I could have allowed myself to be authentic—to be free.

HOW DID I RECOVER FROM THIS?

I recovered by refusing to give up. I held on to the hope that things could get better—*Oh God, please help me get better*. I committed to the work of slowly untangling the knots I'd wrapped myself in over all these years. It took patience, perseverance, and grit to keep going when I wanted to quit, but I knew that happiness and freedom were waiting for me at the end.

And I was right.

DID I LOSE EVERYTHING I WORKED SO HARD FOR?

No. I didn't lose a single thing—except the buried shards and traumas of my past. My wife, children, family, work associates, and friends supported me along the way. I gained stronger, more meaningful relationships, a healthier perspective on life, and a strong desire to help others achieve the same.

AM I A FAILURE FOR SHOWING CRACKS IN MY ARMOR?

No. I am a testament to the strength and resilience of men. We can be severely hurt and go right on fighting for those we love. It wasn't until I allowed myself to truly love Whitney that I found the strength to overcome what had been dragging me under. I am not a failure—I am a miracle.

WHO AM I?

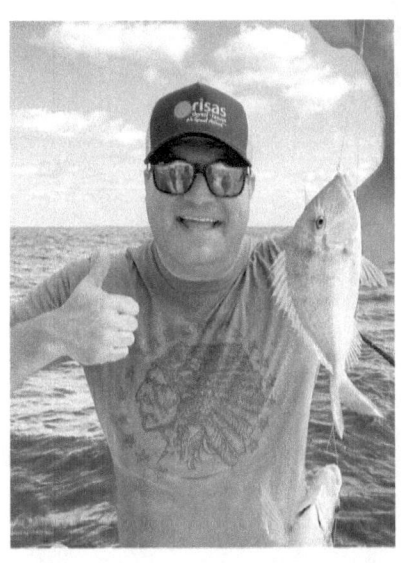

I am many things: a father, husband, business partner, brother, son, mentor, disciple, and student. I am a phoenix reborn from the ashes of my painful past. I am the protector of my inner child, a warrior willing to battle my demons.

I am Whitney Wright, and I couldn't be happier about that.

Thank you for joining me on this journey! I encourage you to reflect on your own experiences and growth and start on your own healing path if needed.

As we continue on this path of healing and growth together, let's hold fast to hope. Let's lean into our own resilience and trust in the incredible power of our stories to change lives and transform the world around us. Because in the end, that's what life is all about—not just surviving, but thriving, and using our experiences to light the way for others who may be struggling in the darkness.

We can make a difference, one story and one boundary at a time.

So let's stay the course, fellow Men Under Pressure—together, we're unstoppable.

For more resources, and to connect on social media, visit *MenUnderPressure.com*.

> **"I don't know where I'm going from here,**
> **but I promise it won't be boring."**
> —DAVID BOWIE

A P P E N D I X   A

QUESTIONNAIRES FOR SELF-REFLECTION AND EXPLORATION

*Remember: This book explicitly does **not** offer medical advice for mental or physical health, and the following questionnaires are not meant to diagnose. Instead, these questionnaires are invitations for you to ask yourself deep questions and self-reflect. Based on the results of any of the questionnaires—or even the feelings taking them may bring up within you—consider consulting with a health professional.*

EXPLORING TOXIC SHAME

Reflect and answer the following questions honestly. Rate each statement based on your experience:

1. Feelings of Worthlessness
   - Do you often feel that you aren't good enough or that you don't deserve love or respect?

2. Self-Criticism
   - Do you frequently criticize yourself or engage in negative self-talk?

3. Hiding or Withdrawing
   - Do you tend to avoid social situations or hide from others because you feel inadequate?

4. Perfectionism
   - Do you set unrealistically high standards for yourself, believing that anything less is a failure?

5. Fear of Judgment
   - Are you overly concerned about what others think of you or how they perceive your actions?

6. Difficulty Accepting Praise
   - Do you struggle to accept compliments or feel uncomfortable when others praise you?

7. Comparison to Others
   - Do you often compare yourself to others and feel like you fall short?

8. Feeling Unlovable
    - Do you believe that there's something fundamentally wrong with you that makes you unlovable?

9. Regret and Guilt
    - Do you frequently dwell on past mistakes or decisions, feeling intense regret or guilt?

10. Overapologizing
    - Do you find yourself apologizing excessively, even when it's not necessary?

11. Avoiding Vulnerability
    - Do you avoid showing vulnerability or expressing your true feelings for fear of being judged?

12. Discomfort with Emotions
    - Do you struggle to express or even acknowledge your emotions, feeling ashamed of them?

After answering these questions, reflect on your responses. Are there specific patterns or themes that emerge? It may be helpful to discuss these feelings with a mental health professional to explore them further.

EXPLORING CHILDHOOD TRAUMA

Reflect on your childhood and answer the following questions honestly. Rate each statement based on your experience:

1. I have memories from my childhood that I can't fully recall or understand.
   - ○ Strongly Disagree
   - ○ Disagree
   - ○ Neutral
   - ○ Agree
   - ○ Strongly Agree

2. Certain situations, places, or people trigger strong emotional reactions or discomfort, but I don't understand why.
   - ○ Strongly Disagree
   - ○ Disagree
   - ○ Neutral
   - ○ Agree
   - ○ Strongly Agree

3. I often feel a sense of unease or anxiety without knowing why.
   - O Strongly Disagree
   - O Disagree
   - O Neutral
   - O Agree
   - O Strongly Agree

4. I've had dreams or nightmares about my childhood that leave me feeling unsettled.
   - O Strongly Disagree
   - O Disagree
   - O Neutral
   - O Agree
   - O Strongly Agree

5. I find it hard to trust others or feel close to people, even those I care about.
   - O Strongly Disagree
   - O Disagree
   - O Neutral
   - O Agree
   - O Strongly Agree

6. I avoid talking about my childhood or feel uncomfortable when others bring it up.
   - O Strongly Disagree
   - O Disagree
   - O Neutral
   - O Agree
   - O Strongly Agree

7. I have feelings of shame or guilt related to my childhood experiences, even if I can't pinpoint why.
   - O Strongly Disagree
   - O Disagree
   - O Neutral
   - O Agree
   - O Strongly Agree

8. I struggle with emotional regulation (e.g., anger, sadness) that seems disproportionate to current situations.
   - O Strongly Disagree
   - O Disagree
   - O Neutral
   - O Agree
   - O Strongly Agree

9. I have difficulty recalling positive memories from my childhood.
   - O Strongly Disagree
   - O Disagree
   - O Neutral
   - O Agree
   - O Strongly Agree

10. I feel like I carry an emotional weight from my childhood that affects my daily life.
    - O Strongly Disagree
    - O Disagree
    - O Neutral
    - O Agree
    - O Strongly Agree

Review your responses. A higher number of "Agree" and "Strongly Agree" answers may suggest the presence of hidden traumatic experiences or unresolved issues from your childhood.

If you find that many of these statements resonate with you, consider reaching out to a mental health professional who can help you explore these feelings and experiences in a safe environment.

EXPLORING CODEPENDENCY

For each statement, please indicate how often you relate to the following behaviors in your relationships:

1. I often feel responsible for other people's feelings and well-being.
   - O Never
   - O Sometimes
   - O Often
   - O Very Often

2. I have trouble setting boundaries with others.
   - O Never
   - O Sometimes
   - O Often
   - O Very Often

3. I frequently prioritize others' needs over my own.
   - O Never
   - O Sometimes
   - O Often
   - O Very Often

4. I feel a sense of guilt or anxiety when I think about saying "no" to someone.
   - O Never
   - O Sometimes
   - O Often
   - O Very Often

5. I often stay in relationships even when they're unhealthy or unfulfilling.
   - O Never
   - O Sometimes
   - O Often
   - O Very Often

6. I find myself trying to fix or rescue others, even at my own expense.
   - O Never
   - O Sometimes
   - O Often
   - O Very Often

7. I feel empty or lost when I'm not in a relationship.
   - O Never
   - O Sometimes
   - O Often
   - O Very Often

8. I often suppress my own feelings and needs to keep the peace in my relationships.
   O Never
   O Sometimes
   O Often
   O Very Often

9. I feel anxious when I'm not needed by others.
   O Never
   O Sometimes
   O Often
   O Very Often

10. I often seek validation or approval from others to feel good about myself.
   O Never
   O Sometimes
   O Often
   O Very Often

Count the number of responses you marked as "Often" and "Very Often." A higher number of affirmative responses may indicate a tendency toward codependency.

If you find that you relate to several of these behaviors, consider reaching out to a mental health professional for guidance and support.

EXPLORING UNHEALTHY COPING MECHANISMS

For each statement, please indicate how often you have engaged in the following behaviors in response to stress or difficult emotions **in the past month**:

1. I often turn to food or binge eating to cope with stress or negative feelings.
   - ○ Never
   - ○ Sometimes
   - ○ Often
   - ○ Very Often

2. I frequently isolate myself from friends or family when I'm feeling overwhelmed.
   - ○ Never
   - ○ Sometimes
   - ○ Often
   - ○ Very Often

3. I find myself using alcohol, drugs, or other substances to escape from my problems.
   - ○ Never
   - ○ Sometimes
   - ○ Often
   - ○ Very Often

4. I often engage in excessive shopping or spending to feel better.
   - O Never
   - O Sometimes
   - O Often
   - O Very Often

5. I frequently procrastinate or avoid responsibilities when I feel stressed.
   - O Never
   - O Sometimes
   - O Often
   - O Very Often

6. I often express my feelings through anger or irritability rather than addressing them directly.
   - O Never
   - O Sometimes
   - O Often
   - O Very Often

7. I find myself engaging in self-harm or other risky behaviors to cope with emotional pain.
   - O Never
   - O Sometimes
   - O Often
   - O Very Often

8. I frequently rely on distractions, like binge-watching TV or scrolling through social media, to avoid dealing with my emotions.
   - O Never
   - O Sometimes
   - O Often
   - O Very Often

9. I often feel compelled to please others at the expense of my own needs and feelings.
   - O Never
   - O Sometimes
   - O Often
   - O Very Often

10. I frequently downplay my feelings or convince myself that I shouldn't feel the way I do.
    - O Never
    - O Sometimes
    - O Often
    - O Very Often

Count the number of responses you marked as "Often" and "Very Often." A higher number of affirmative responses may indicate a tendency toward unhealthy coping mechanisms.

If you find that you relate to several of these behaviors, consider reaching out to a mental health professional for guidance and support.

EXPLORING ADHD

For each statement, please indicate how often you have experienced the following **in the past six months**:

1. I often have trouble paying attention to details and make careless mistakes in my work or other activities.
   - O Never
   - O Occasionally
   - O Frequently
   - O Very Often

2. I find it difficult to pay attention during tasks or activities.
   - O Never
   - O Occasionally
   - O Frequently
   - O Very Often

3. I often fail to notice when I'm being spoken to directly.
   - O Never
   - O Occasionally
   - O Frequently
   - O Very Often

4. I frequently do not follow through on instructions and fail to finish schoolwork, chores, or duties.
   - O Never
   - O Occasionally
   - O Frequently
   - O Very Often

5. I often have trouble organizing tasks and activities.
   - O Never
   - O Occasionally
   - O Frequently
   - O Very Often

6. I often avoid or dislike tasks that require sustained mental effort.
   - O Never
   - O Occasionally
   - O Frequently
   - O Very Often

7. I frequently lose things necessary for tasks and activities (e.g., keys, glasses, paperwork).
   - O Never
   - O Occasionally
   - O Frequently
   - O Very Often

8. I'm easily distracted by extraneous stimuli or unrelated thoughts.
    - O Never
    - O Occasionally
    - O Frequently
    - O Very Often

9. I often forget to do daily activities (e.g., chores, errands).
    - O Never
    - O Occasionally
    - O Frequently
    - O Very Often

10. I often fidget or tap my hands or feet, or squirm in my seat.
    - O Never
    - O Occasionally
    - O Frequently
    - O Very Often

11. I frequently leave my seat in situations where remaining seated is expected.
    - O Never
    - O Occasionally
    - O Frequently
    - O Very Often

12. I often talk excessively or interrupt others.
    O Never
    O Occasionally
    O Frequently
    O Very Often

Count the number of responses you marked as "Frequently" and "Very Often." A higher number of affirmative responses may indicate a higher likelihood of ADHD symptoms.

If you identify with several of these symptoms frequently, consider consulting a healthcare professional for further evaluation and support.

EXPLORING PTSD

Reflect and answer the following questions honestly:

1. Traumatic Events
   • Have you experienced or witnessed a traumatic event that felt overwhelming or life-threatening?

2. Intrusive Memories
   • Do you frequently have distressing memories or flashbacks of the traumatic event(s) that disrupt your daily life?

3. Nightmares
   - Do you experience recurrent nightmares related to the traumatic event(s)?

4. Avoidance
   - Do you avoid reminders, people, places, or activities that trigger memories of the traumatic experience?

5. Emotional Numbness
   - Do you feel emotionally numb or detached from others, making it difficult to connect with friends or loved ones?

6. Hyperarousal
   - Do you often feel on edge, easily startled, or hypervigilant, as if you're always anticipating danger?

7. Irritability and Anger
   - Have you noticed increased irritability or anger, including outbursts that seem disproportionate to the situation?

8. Concentration Difficulties
   - Do you find it hard to concentrate or focus on tasks, often feeling overwhelmed by distractions?

9. Changes in Mood
   - Have you experienced significant changes in your mood, such as feelings of hopelessness, sadness, or anxiety?

10. Physical Symptoms
    - Do you experience physical symptoms such as headaches, stomachaches, or other unexplained pain, especially in relation to stress?

11. Substance Use
    - Have you turned to alcohol, drugs, or other substances as a way to cope with your feelings or memories related to the trauma?

12. Social Withdrawal
    - Have you withdrawn from friends, family, or activities that you once enjoyed?

After completing this questionnaire, consider how these symptoms may be impacting your life. If you resonate with several of these questions, it might be beneficial to seek support from a mental health professional who specializes in trauma and PTSD.

EXPLORING ADRENAL FATIGUE

For each statement, please indicate how often you have experienced the following **in the past month**:

1. I often feel tired or fatigued, even after a full night's sleep.
    - O Not at all
    - O A little
    - O Somewhat
    - O Very often

2. I struggle to get out of bed in the morning, feeling unrefreshed.
    - O Not at all
    - O A little
    - O Somewhat
    - O Very often

3. I have difficulty concentrating or remembering things.
    - O Not at all
    - O A little
    - O Somewhat
    - O Very often

4. I feel overwhelmed by stress more than I used to.
    - O Not at all
    - O A little
    - O Somewhat
    - O Very often

5. I crave caffeine or sugary foods to help boost my energy.
   - O Not at all
   - O A little
   - O Somewhat
   - O Very often

6. I experience mood swings or irritability.
   - O Not at all
   - O A little
   - O Somewhat
   - O Very often

7. I have frequent headaches or migraines.
   - O Not at all
   - O A little
   - O Somewhat
   - O Very often

8. I feel an increased need for sleep but still wake up feeling tired.
   - O Not at all
   - O A little
   - O Somewhat
   - O Very often

9. I have a lower tolerance for stress than I used to.
   - O Not at all
   - O A little
   - O Somewhat
   - O Very often

10. I find myself feeling less motivated or less engaged in daily activities.
    - O Not at all
    - O A little
    - O Somewhat
    - O Very often

Count the number of responses you marked as "Somewhat" and "Very often." A higher number of affirmative responses may indicate a higher level of adrenal fatigue.

If you identify with several of these symptoms frequently, consider seeking advice from a healthcare professional for further evaluation and support.

EXPLORING DEPRESSION

For each statement, please indicate how often you have experienced the following **in the past two weeks**:

1. I feel sad or hopeless.
   - O Not at all
   - O Several days
   - O More than half the days
   - O Nearly every day

2. I have little interest or pleasure in doing things I usually enjoy.
   - O Not at all
   - O Several days
   - O More than half the days
   - O Nearly every day

3. I have trouble sleeping or sleep too much.
   - O Not at all
   - O Several days
   - O More than half the days
   - O Nearly every day

4. I feel tired or have little energy.
   - O Not at all
   - O Several days
   - O More than half the days
   - O Nearly every day

5. I have a poor appetite or tend to overeat.
   - O Not at all
   - O Several days
   - O More than half the days
   - O Nearly every day

6. I feel bad about myself or think that I'm a failure.
   - O Not at all
   - O Several days
   - O More than half the days
   - O Nearly every day

7. I have trouble concentrating on things, such as reading or watching television.
   - O Not at all
   - O Several days
   - O More than half the days
   - O Nearly every day

8. I sometimes think I'd be better off dead or consider hurting myself in some way.
   - O Not at all
   - O Several days
   - O More than half the days
   - O Nearly every day

Count the number of responses you marked as "More than half the days" and "Nearly every day." A higher number of affirmative responses may indicate a higher level of depression.

If you find that you are experiencing several of these symptoms frequently, consider reaching out to a mental health professional for further evaluation and support.

EXPLORING ANXIETY

For each statement, please indicate how often you have experienced the following **in the past two weeks**:

1. I feel restless or on edge.
   - O Not at all
   - O Several days
   - O More than half the days
   - O Nearly every day

2. I find it difficult to relax or calm down.
   - O Not at all
   - O Several days
   - O More than half the days
   - O Nearly every day

3. I worry excessively about different aspects of my life (e.g., work, health, relationships).
   - O Not at all
   - O Several days
   - O More than half the days
   - O Nearly every day

4. I have trouble concentrating or my mind goes blank.
   - O Not at all
   - O Several days
   - O More than half the days
   - O Nearly every day

5. I feel easily fatigued or worn out.
   - O Not at all
   - O Several days
   - O More than half the days
   - O Nearly every day

6. I experience muscle tension or physical discomfort.
   - O Not at all
   - O Several days
   - O More than half the days
   - O Nearly every day

7. I find myself avoiding certain situations due to anxiety.
    - ○ Not at all
    - ○ Several days
    - ○ More than half the days
    - ○ Nearly every day

8. I feel overwhelmed by feelings of fear or dread.
    - ○ Not at all
    - ○ Several days
    - ○ More than half the days
    - ○ Nearly every day

Count the number of responses you marked as "More than half the days" and "Nearly every day." A higher number of affirmative responses may indicate a higher level of anxiety.

If you find that you are experiencing several of these symptoms frequently, consider reaching out to a mental health professional for further evaluation and support.

EXPLORING BURNOUT

For each statement, please indicate how often you have experienced the following **in the past month**:

1. I feel emotionally drained from my work or daily responsibilities.
   - O Not at all
   - O A little
   - O Somewhat
   - O Very often

2. I've become more cynical or negative about my job or responsibilities.
   - O Not at all
   - O A little
   - O Somewhat
   - O Very often

3. I lack motivation or enthusiasm for my work.
   - O Not at all
   - O A little
   - O Somewhat
   - O Very often

4. I find it difficult to concentrate on tasks.
   - O Not at all
   - O A little
   - O Somewhat
   - O Very often

5. I feel overwhelmed by my workload.
   - O Not at all
   - O A little
   - O Somewhat
   - O Very often

6. I feel detached or disconnected from my work or colleagues.
   - O Not at all
   - O A little
   - O Somewhat
   - O Very often

7. I often feel stressed or anxious about my responsibilities.
   - O Not at all
   - O A little
   - O Somewhat
   - O Very often

8. I have physical symptoms of stress (e.g., headaches, stomach issues, fatigue).
   - O Not at all
   - O A little
   - O Somewhat
   - O Very often

Count the number of responses you marked as "Somewhat" and "Very often." A higher number of affirmative responses may indicate a higher level of burnout.

If you identify with several of these symptoms frequently, consider seeking support from a mental health professional or exploring strategies for managing burnout.

EXPLORING ADDICTION

Reflect and answer the following questions honestly:

1. Compulsive Behavior
   - Do you find yourself engaging in certain behaviors or using substances even when you don't want to?

2. Loss of Control
   - Have you tried to cut down or stop using a substance or behavior but found it difficult to do so?

3. Neglecting Responsibilities
   - Have you neglected important responsibilities at work, home, or school due to substance abuse or engaging in certain behaviors?

4. Preoccupation
   - Do you spend a lot of time thinking about, obtaining, or recovering from the effects of a substance or behavior?

5. Withdrawal Symptoms
   - Do you experience physical or emotional withdrawal symptoms (like anxiety, irritability, or cravings) when you try to reduce or stop using a substance?

6. Escalating Use
   - Have you noticed that you need to use more of a substance or engage in a behavior more frequently to achieve the same effect?

7. Risky Situations
   - Do you engage in risky behaviors or find yourself in dangerous situations as a result of your addiction?

8. Isolation
   - Have you withdrawn from friends, family, or activities you once enjoyed in favor of using substances or engaging in addictive behaviors?

9. Denial
   - Do you find it hard to acknowledge the negative impact of your addiction on your life or the lives of others?

10. Attempts to Hide Use
   - Do you go out of your way to hide your substance use or addictive behaviors from others?

11. Continued Use Despite Consequences
   - Do you continue to use substances or engage in behaviors even after experiencing negative consequences (health issues, legal problems, relationship troubles)?

12. Emotional Regulation
   - Do you use substances or engage in behaviors to cope with stress, anxiety, or other emotional issues?

A higher number of affirmative responses may indicate a higher sensitivity to addiction. If you identify with several of these symptoms frequently, consider seeking support from a mental health professional and/or exploring strategies for mitigation.

EXPLORING MENTAL HEALTH RESOURCES
AND SUPPORT OPTIONS

If you're struggling with mental health issues, know that help is available. Here's a list of resources in the United States that can provide support:

- National Suicide Prevention Lifeline
    - Call 1-800-273-8255 (Available 24/7)
    - Website: https://988lifeline.org

- Crisis Text Line
    - Text HOME to 741741 (Available 24/7)
    - Website: crisistextline.org

- National Alliance on Mental Illness (NAMI)
    - Helpline: 1-800-950-NAMI (6264)
    - Website: nami.org
    - Offers support groups, education programs, and advocacy

- Substance Abuse and Mental Health Services Administration (SAMHSA)
    - National Helpline: 1-800-662-HELP (4357)
    - Website: samhsa.gov
    - Provides referrals to local treatment facilities, support groups, and community-based organizations

ONLINE THERAPY PLATFORMS

- BetterHelp: betterhelp.com
- Talkspace: talkspace.com

MENTAL HEALTH APPS

- Calm: Meditation and sleep app
- Headspace: Mindfulness and meditation app
- Moodfit: Mood tracking and mental health tools
- Insight Timer: Hundreds of free guided meditations

ONLINE COMMUNITIES

- Reddit's r/mentalhealth: reddit.com/r/mentalhealth
- 7 Cups: 7cups.com—Free emotional support and online therapy

LOCAL RESOURCES

- Community Mental Health Centers: Search for centers in your area
- University Counseling Centers: For students, check your school's website
- Employee Assistance Programs (EAPs): Check with your employer about available mental health services

APPENDIX B
RECOMMENDED READING

For further self-reflection and exploration, I recommend the following:

- *Guilt & Shame: Masters of Disguise* by Jane Middelton-Moz
- *Mine Are Too: A Children's Guide To Divorce* by Spencer Caldwell
- *Driven to Distraction: Recognizing and Coping with Attention Deficit Disorder from Childhood Through Adulthood* by Dr. Edward Hallowell and Dr. John Ratey
- *ADHD 2.0: New Science and Essential Strategies for Thriving with Distraction* by Dr. Edward Hallowell and Dr. John Ratey
- *The Total Money Makeover* by Dave Ramsey
- *Burnout Proof* by Michael Levitt
- *No More Mr. Nice Guy* by Dr. Robert Glover

- *His Needs, Her Needs: Building a Marriage That Lasts* by Dr. Willard F. Harley Jr.
- *12 Rules for Life: An Antidote for Chaos* by Jordan B. Peterson
- *Essentialism* by Greg McKeown
- *Boundaries: When to Say Yes, How to Say No to Take Control of Your Life* by Dr. Henry Cloud and Dr. John Townsend
- *The Gifts of Imperfection: Let Go of Who You Think You're Supposed to Be and Embrace Who You Are* by Brené Brown (and the rest of her impressive catalogue!)
- *The Power of Now* by Eckhart Tolle
- *Start with Why* by Simon Sinek
- *Getting Past Your Past: Take Control of Your Life With Self-Help Techniques from EMDR Therapy* by Dr. Francine Shapiro
- *The Body Keeps the Score: Brain, Mind, and Body in the Healing of Trauma* by Dr. Bessel van der Kolk

UNLOCK THE BONUS CHAPTER

30 YEARS OF ANXIETY, GONE IN 30 SECONDS

There was one story we couldn't fit inside this
book—but it's too powerful not to share.
In this bonus chapter, Whitney reveals the
breakthrough moment that changed everything
after decades of anxiety, panic, and PTSD.

Get access to the full story now:
Scan the QR code or visit
bonus.menunderpressure.com.

Who knows, this chapter could change your life too.

NOTES

1 "Mental Illness," National Institute of Mental Health, last updated September 2024, https://www.nimh.nih.gov/health/statistics/mental-illness.

2 Remember: This book explicitly does not offer medical advice for mental or physical health, and these questionnaires are not meant to diagnose. Instead, these questionnaires are invitations for you to ask yourself deep questions and self-reflect. Based on the results of any of the questionnaires—or even the feelings taking them may bring up within you—consider consulting with a health professional.

3 National Institute of Mental Health, "Mental Health."

4 For a self-reflection questionnaire on toxic shame, refer to Appendix A.

5 For a self-reflection questionnaire on childhood trauma, refer to Appendix A.

6 For a self-reflection questionnaire on codependency, refer to Appendix A.

7 "Codependency," Psychology Today, accessed February 13, 2025, https://www.psychologytoday.com/intl/basics/codependency.

8 For a self-reflection questionnaire on unhealthy coping mechanisms, refer to Appendix A.

9 Kathleen A. Ports et al., "Adverse Childhood Experiences and Sexual Victimization in Adulthood," *Child Abuse & Neglect* 51 (2016): 313–22, accessed February 13, 2025, https://doi.org/10.1016/j.chiabu.2015.08.017.

10 For a self-reflection questionnaire on ADHD, refer to Appendix A.

11 Louise C. Druedahl and Sofia Kälvemark Sporrong, "Managing Complexity: Exploring Decision Making on Medication by Young Adults with ADHD," *Pharmacy* 6, no. 2 (2018): 33, accessed February 13, 2025, https://doi.org/10.3390/pharmacy6020033.

12 J.R.R. Tolkien, *The Fellowship of the Ring* (George Allen & Unwin, 1954).

13 João M. Carvalho Fernando et al., "Emotion Regulation and Excessive Aggression: The Role of Child Maltreatment," *European Journal of Psychotraumatology* 5 (2014): 1–10, accessed February 13, 2025, https://pubmed.ncbi.nlm.nih.gov/24283697/.

14 Vincent J. Felitti et al., "Relationship of Childhood Abuse and Household Dysfunction to Many of the Leading Causes of Death in Adults: The Adverse Childhood Experiences (ACE) Study," *American Journal of Preventive Medicine* 14, no. 4 (1998): 245–258, accessed February 13, 2025, https://pubmed.ncbi.nlm.nih.gov/9635069/.

15 Pauline R. Clance and Suzanne A. Imes, "The Impostor Phenomenon in High Achieving Women: Dynamics and Therapeutic Intervention," *Psychotherapy: Theory, Research & Practice* 15, no. 3 (1978): 241–247.

16 Bessel van der Kolk, *The Body Keeps the Score: Brain, Mind, and Body in the Healing of Trauma* (Viking, 2014).

17 For a self-reflection questionnaire on PTSD, refer to Appendix A.

18 Lisa M. Shin and Israel Liberzon, "The Neurocircuitry of Fear, Stress, and Anxiety Disorders," *Neuropsychopharmacology* 35, no. 1 (2010): 169–191, https://doi.org/10.1038/npp.2009.83.

19 Scott L. Rauch et al., "Neurocircuitry Models of Posttraumatic Stress Disorder and Extinction: Human Neuroimaging Research—Past, Present, and Future," *Biological Psychiatry* 60, no. 4 (2006): 376–382, https://doi.org/10.1016/j.biopsych.2006.06.004.

20 For a self-reflection questionnaire on adrenal fatigue, refer to Appendix A.

21 Genovino Ferri, "Contemporary Reichian Analysis: Evolutive Stage, Epigenetics, and the Neuromediator Dynamic," *Psychotherapy Today* 14, no. 1 (2024): 19–29, https://somaticpsychotherapytoday.com/wp-content/uploads/2024/05/Contemporary-Reichian-Analysis-by-Genovino-Ferri-May-2024.pdf.

22 "Lifestyle Changes for Shifting Cortisol Levels," The Institute for Functional Medicine, last updated June 28, 2021, https://www.ifm.org/articles/lifestyle-changes-for-cortisol.

23 Gabrielle Salvatore et al., "Psychosocial Stress and Cardiovascular Risk: State of the Science and Areas for Attention," *Outlook*, 2024. https://www.sbm.org/publications/outlook/issues/fall-2024/psychosocial-stress-and-cardiovascular-risk-state-of-the-science-and-areas-for-attention/full-article.

24 For a self-reflection questionnaire on depression, refer to Appendix A.

25 For a self-reflection questionnaire on anxiety, refer to Appendix A.

26 "Depression," National Institute of Mental Health, last reviewed February 2025, https://www.nimh.nih.gov/health/publications/men-and-depression.

27 "Suicide Statistics," American Foundation for Suicide Prevention, accessed February 13, 2025, https://afsp.org/suicide-statistics/.

28 G.A.H. Guevara et al., "Cardiovascular Risk Estimation and the Role of Anxiety in Emotional Wellbeing," *Journal of General Medicine* (2025), accessed February 16, 2025.

29 Marc Dörner et al., "Cross-Sectional Study on the Impact of Adverse Childhood Experiences on Psychological Distress in Patients with Implantable Cardioverter-Defibrillators," *Journal of Psychosomatic Research* (2025), accessed February 16, 2025, https://doi.org/10.1016/j.jpsychores.2024.112033.

30 Maria Picó-Pérez et al., "Neural Predictors of Cognitive-Behavioral Therapy Outcome in Anxiety-Related Disorders: A Meta-Analysis of Task-Based fMRI Studies," *Psychological Medicine* (2022), accessed February 11, 2025, https://www.doctortic.net/CBCN2023/2023_Fullana_2022.pdf.

31 For a self-reflection questionnaire on burnout, refer to Appendix A.

32 "Dental Education," American Dental Association, accessed February 13, 2025, https://www.ada.org/resources/research/health-policy-institute/dental-education.

33 "Member Data," American Association of Orthodontists, accessed February 13, 2025, https://www2.aaoinfo.org/membership/member-data/.

34 Understanding these tendencies is the first step toward addressing and managing people-pleasing behaviors. While this section of the book focuses on self-improvement without therapy, it's important to consider seeking professional help if you identify as codependent or a people pleaser. Professional guidance can provide deeper insights into the root causes of these behaviors.

35 Henry Cloud and John Townsend, *Boundaries: When to Say Yes, How to Say No to Take Control of Your Life* (Zondervan, 1992).

36 Brené Brown, *The Gifts of Imperfection: Let Go of Who You Think You're Supposed to Be and Embrace Who You Are* (Hazelden Publishing, 2010).

37 For a self-reflection questionnaire on addiction, refer to Appendix A.

38 "Only 1 in 5 US Adults with Opioid Use Disorder Received Medications to Treat It in 2021," National Institute on Drug Abuse, August 7, 2023, https://nida.nih.gov/news-events/news-releases/2023/08/only-1-in-5-us-adults-with-opioid-use-disorder-received-medications-to-treat-it-in-2021.

ACKNOWLEDGEMENTS

Congratulations on completing my manly mental health recovery guide! My ultimate aim in writing this book was to help you improve your life—or the life of someone you care about—and I sincerely hope I've achieved that.

First and foremost, my deepest gratitude goes to my amazing wife, Margaret. You are not only the love of my life but also my best friend. Without your wisdom, thoughtful editing, and unwavering encouragement, this book might have remained nothing more than a pipe dream. Your steadfast compassion and love have kept me from crumbling under the weight of it all. I am, now and always, eternally yours.

To my three incredible children—affectionately known in our home as Moose, Lemon, and Twink—thank you for standing by me through every high and low. Your hugs, kind words, vibrant personalities, and perfectly timed jokes have kept me grounded. I love you with all my heart, and being your dad is the greatest privilege of my life.

A heartfelt thank you to my parents, siblings, and all my wonderful in-laws. Your enduring love and support over the years mean the world to me. And a special thanks to Grandpa Jay for teaching me the art of storytelling and for showing me how to fish so well that I could catch fish even on a dusty road.

Thank you to the extraordinary doctors, therapists, and staff at Sierra Tucson. Maureen O'Connor-Strout, your kindness, dedication, and expertise with EMDR have transformed my life—I will forever be grateful. Bill Reynolds, your guidance in helping patients heal is nothing short of miraculous. Thank you both.

A huge shout-out to my editors—Lisa Caskey, Jessica Burdg, and Samantha Hendrix—and to my publishing and marketing team, including Dan Curran, John Ayers, Deborah Iddon, and Darnah Mercieca. Without your guidance, I'd still be lost in the labyrinth of self-publishing. Thank you also, Jessica Kleinman, for offering me an insider's look into the world of publishing.

As the saying goes, "It takes a village to raise a child," and the same is true for writing a book. I am deeply grateful to the many Men Under Pressure who courageously shared their stories, allowing me to pass them on to you. Your bravery and selfless-ness will always hold a special place in my heart.

An enormous thank you to my beta readers—Margaret Wright, Justin Wright, Kristen "Kris" Machain, Nick Gardner, Austin Smith, and Lonnie Ruscito. Your feedback on the first draft was instrumental in shaping this book. Special thanks, too, to my brothers from Sierra Tucson—known as Low T, Old Fat Baldwin, and Pablo Escobar—for always being there when I needed you most, and to Kenny G. for the advice that sparked my journey into writing. I also want to honor two fallen warriors I met at Sierra Tucson, known as John Wick and Johnny SmallCuff. The weight of past traumas took two beautiful souls far too soon, and their loss pains my heart. I miss you, my brothers.

To my psychiatrist, Dr. Saba Monsoor, thank you for gently pushing me forward with kindness and encouragement. I also want to acknowledge the talented therapists—Judy Steenblik, Robin Goldstein, and Cody Weldon—whose guidance has been invaluable. And to my naturopathic doctor, Dr. John Robinson, thank you for helping me balance my body's systems and hormones.

I also want to express my gratitude to a few remarkably talented men whose books and unforgettable protagonists impacted me during my darkest struggles. Your works provided comfort, strength, and the courage to write my own story.

- Brandon Sanderson, thank you for The Stormlight Archive. Kaladin and Bridge Four taught me about resilience, camaraderie, and perseverance. The Cosmere is a gift, and I hope someday to meet Wit—a character whose name I truly admire.

- To the late Robert Jordan, thank you for The Wheel of Time. While Rand al'Thor inspired me, it was Mat Cauthon's irrepressible antics that brightened my darkest days, showing me that heroes aren't born—they are forged in the furnace of adversity.

- Patrick Rothfuss, thank you for The Kingkiller Chronicle. Your lyrical prose is so beautiful that I will always long to sit with Kvothe at the Waystone Inn, listening to his adventures—and perhaps even learning the name of the wind.

To my friends and colleagues who have supported me—not only on this healing journey but throughout my entire life—I am deeply grateful. A heartfelt thank you goes to the Jim and Mary Jane Robbins family; without your unwavering support during my challenging teenage years, I truly don't know where I would be today.

Finally, may this guide bring hope and healing to those who need it most. Though I may no longer fix smiles with my hands, through my words I hope to restore a lost smile to the face of a Man Under Pressure.

www.ingramcontent.com/pod-product-compliance
Lightning Source LLC
Chambersburg PA
CBHW021217130626
46554CB00004B/1253